# SWORDS OF TRUTH

## Basics of Fencing & Character Development

THANK YOU FOR BEING PART OF THE FENCING CLASS. I JUST WANTED TO SHARE THIS BOOK WITH YOU AND SPEAK A BLESSING OVER YOU. "THE LORD BLESS YOU AND KEEP YOU; THE LORD MAKE HIS FACE SHINE ON YOU AND BE GRACIOUS TO YOU; THE LORD TURN HIS FACE TOWARD YOU AND GIVE YOU PEACE."

NUMBERS 6:24-26

[illegible signature]

# SWORDS OF TRUTH

## Basics of Fencing & Character Development

by

Sir Kyle Wilder

First Edition: 03-2018
Printed in the United States of America
ISBN: 9781642547566

# Dedication

I would like to give all the credit for this book to my Lord and Savior Jesus Christ. Jesus has given me some great relationships with many people who have believed in my abilities and in me: My loving wife Stacy, who has always been in my corner. My daughter Ana, who has shared her daddy with so many. My second mom Bonnie, a true friend and my editor. Pastors Alan and Cherie, who have given me their love, support and guidance, along with Restoration Life Church family. Andrea V., our future "Dr. Ducky". My friend and instructor, Maestro Craig, and the Tri-Blade Fencing group.

# TABLE OF CONTENTS

TABLE OF CONTENTS ............................................. vi
PREFACE ..................................................................... ix

KNIGHTLY VALUES ................................................. 1
Compassion ................................................................. 4
Kindness / Sportsmanship ............................................ 8
Humility ..................................................................... 13
Quiet Strength / Gentleness ......................................... 18
Discipline ................................................................... 23
Imposed Discipline .................................................. 24
Self-Discipline ......................................................... 26
True discipline ......................................................... 28
Even-Tempered ........................................................... 31
Content ....................................................................... 38
Forgive ....................................................................... 42

FENCING FOUNDATIONS & SKILLS .................... 47
Safety ......................................................................... 48
Parts of the Foil .......................................................... 50
The Hilt .................................................................... 50
The Blade ................................................................. 51
Foil, Epee, and Saber ............................................... 52
En Garde / Advance / Retreat ..................................... 53
En Garde .................................................................. 53
Advance ................................................................... 53
Retreat ..................................................................... 55
Lunge / Recover .......................................................... 56
Target Areas ............................................................... 58
"Right-of-Way" or Priority ....................................... 59
Inside / Outside Line ................................................... 60
Parries ........................................................................ 63
Coupé / Disengage ...................................................... 65

Semaphores ........ 67
Judging a Bout ........ 72
Appendix A ........ 75
Appendix B ........ 78
Glossary of Fencing Terms ........ 78
Appendix C ........ 84
Partial list of Feeling words ........ 84

KNIGHTLY VALUES WORKSHEETS ........ 85
Compassion Worksheet ........ 87
Kindness Worksheet ........ 89
Humility Worksheet ........ 91
Quiet Strength Worksheet ........ 93
Discipline Worksheet ........ 95
Even-Tempered Worksheet ........ 97
Content Worksheet ........ 99
Forgiveness Worksheet ........ 101

# PREFACE

When God gives you the opportunity to blend your love of fencing with your passion for developing positive character in this up and coming generation, it gives you a unique community outreach opportunity we called SWORDS OF TRUTH.

My wife and I have been working with young people at Restoration Life Church, Battle Creek, Michigan for many years. Starting in children's ministry and following them on as they grew, to pastor them in youth ministry. We had the opportunity to obtain our Associate Ministers license with Christian International.

We both have a strong passion to see young people develop into who God created them to be, and fulfill their unique destinies, to become assets to the kingdom of God within their communities, cities, states, and nation.

Years ago, we began fencing as a hobby, for a recreational exercise to do as a couple. We fell in love with the sport and much more so, with the positive effect it was having on the young people participating in the fencing club.

Fencing is an honor-based sport with strong historical heritage. Fencing re-introduces, re-enforces and restores positive character traits within the participants. These same character traits also parallel Godly character.

Even within the public school environment, I have seen the traits of honor, integrity, and gratitude transform whole classes of juniors and seniors. In the beginning of a trimester, the students ignore or deny when a point is scored (touche`). By the time we are half-way through the trimester, I do not even have the chance to call the point (touche`) before they are already congratulating their opponent. These are the same character traits we all desire to see cultivated in our generations and communities.

God then gave us a vision in how we can merge these two passions, to be able to reach outside the four walls of our church and affect change in our community. I wanted to give the new fencing students a step-by-step instructional flyer for practicing the newly learned moves. So, I began to write and draw out the needed images.

We started our first pilot session with a small group from the church neighborhood and without the desired flyer. We brought them together once-a-week for an hour-and-a-half of fencing instruction. Fifteen to twenty minutes of that time is set aside for character development discussions with bits of fencing history incorporated along the way. During the pilot session, God began giving me more to write. My flyer is looking more like a book. This Book.

# KNIGHTLY VALUES

Have you ever been on the playground and there is that one kid making fun, picking on or even hurting someone? You may have even joined in so that the bully wouldn't turn it on you. You may have just walked away or you might even have been the one who was being picked on. In all these cases, you know it is wrong!

**WHY?** You might ask. Why are some people like this?

**Lack of Character…** We are to always be working on who we are, trying to make ourselves better. The only thing you can change in the above playground example is you. There is no magic we can use that *"can make others change"*. We can only change ourselves and we can do that by working on our character, which can also have an influence on others.

**What is Character?**

Character is like a GPS unit in a car. As you're going down the road, you have choices. You can turn, go straight or turn around. The GPS is there to let you know if you have turned the wrong way. The GPS might say, "Recalculation" or "Make a Legal U-Turn" to help you get back going the right way. Your GPS will be no good if you don't charge or plug it in. Working on your character is like plugging in your internal GPS.

Compassion
Kindness
Humility
Quiet Strength
Discipline
Even-Tempered
Content
Forgiving

As part of this fencing program, we will help you to work on your character, so that you too, can make the right choices in your school, neighborhood and family.

During the time of the Middle Ages, a list of values (character traits) were attributed to being a knight. The list was never written, and different knightly realms followed different values. Hundreds of years later, people have tried to recreate these lists, but no one really knows exactly what they were.

I have looked at many of these recreated "knightly values" lists. But, in all my searching, I have found that the Bible is the reference that sums them up. The Message Version Bible says it best:

> So, chosen by God for this new life of love, dress in the wardrobe God picked out for you: **compassion**, **kindness**, **humility**, **quiet strength**, **discipline**. Be **even-tempered**, **content** with second place, quick to **forgive** an offense. Forgive as quickly and completely as the Master forgave you. And regardless of what else you put on, wear love. It's your basic, all-purpose garment. Never be without it.
>
> ~ Bible Colossians 3:12-14
>
> The Message (bold added)

In walking out these values, love is formed. The values are the threads that make up the clothing of Love. Let's look at these values. First, you'll see Googles definition of the values, second some biblical examples, and finally examples of how I have walked them out in addition to some ideas to help you to walk them out as well.

## COMPASSION

com·pas·sion (kəmˈpaSHən) noun

Concern for the sufferings or misfortunes of others

~ Google

Be kind and compassionate to one another, forgiving each other, just as in Christ, God forgave you.

~ Bible Ephesians 4:32 NIV

As a father has compassion on his children, so the LORD has compassion on those who fear him;

~ Bible Psalm 103:13 NIV

When you see someone suffering or mistreated, do you feel badly for that person? Then YOU have compassion. Back to our playground example: If we have true compassion for the person(s) being mistreated, we would not join in, or allow it to continue. We would let an adult know.

We have all seen compassion displayed on the news; when a natural disaster, tragic shooting, etc. occurs in the world, we see many people helping those who are suffering. We have entire organizations that are designed and developed around compassionate assistance, like the American Red Cross, Salvation Army, and The United Way to name a few. You can Google their mission statements and see that their main desire is to help people in hard situations. These organizations have also created in our communities a type of "double-edged sword". People remove themselves from getting involved in other's situations by saying to themselves, "That's why I give to these organizations." It removes their responsibility to show compassion directly to people in their communities.

When I was 14 or 15 years old, my family lived at a local campground for the whole summer. My father would leave every morning to go to work. One stormy morning shortly after he, and other families left for work, we had a tornado come through. We had trees falling everywhere. One tree almost hit my family's camper. Another tree went through the roof of another family's camper and crushed my friend's foot. Once the storm was over, people were coming out of their campers and the tornado shelters to survey the damages.

As we looked around, we noticed that there were very few men left in the campground. The entire campground was without power because two large trees fell across the power lines, phone lines and the only driveway leading in or out of the campground. We could not call anyone for help. It was in the late 70's and cell phones were not widely used yet. So none of the family members who left earlier that morning knew what had happened or what damage there was.

A few men and one nurse, who also stayed the summer at the campground, were inside my friend's camper, freeing his crushed foot. Once they had him freed and loaded into a pick-up truck, the next problem situation was even more evident: getting him to the main road, and in turn to the hospital. The downed trees across the driveway blocked our exit route and heavy woods surrounded the rest of the campground. One of my friends knew a way through the woods. He had hunted in those woods with family for years and we all played games out there.

As my friend guided the truck out of the campground, we turned our attention to clearing the driveway with only a few men present and ten to fifteen youth. The men taught the older teens how to use chain saws and drive the tractors and carts. We went from site to site helping the adults clear out the branches and debris.

Some of the campers were equipped with generators; these families stored all the perishable food. These campsites became the central point for the busy day; serving breakfast, lunch, and dinner for all, providing a cool place for the senior adults, and a place for all to take breaks and get cold drinks.

We pulled together, worked together, and ate together, making sure everyone's needs were met. When my dad and everyone else's family members came home seeing and hearing of all that had happened, they were surprised and proud of how all the youth worked together with compassion for each other.

Compassion will always put others' needs before our own. The world says "live by the Golden Rule: Do unto others as you would have them do unto you." The Bible also says it this way: "love your neighbor as yourself". In today's generation, these rules seem harder and harder to follow. The media, advertising and movies tell us: "Have it your way!", "Just Do It!", and "Show me the Money!" It is all about self, and what is in it for me! They forget to ask themselves, "How can I love my neighbor?" Without compassion, we are not able to love.

Compassion develops in the heart and is an internal value; other people can't see what is happening in your heart. The Bible states that only God knows our heart. King David is a great example of not being able to see what is happening in another person's heart. David broke many of God's rules, but God still said this about David, "I have found David, son of Jesse, a man after my own heart; he will do everything I want him to do." Acts 13:22 NIV.

God has a heart of compassion. That is why He made provision for us to be able to come to him. “For God so loved the world that he gave his one and only Son, that whoever believes in him shall not perish, but have eternal life.” John 3:16 (NIV). In addition, Jesus was moved with compassion, when he healed those who were sick. We should also be moved with compassion and do what we can for others.

**You are Challenged to A Duel!**

In the back of this book, there are a couple questions and a knightly value challenge.

## KINDNESS / SPORTSMANSHIP

kind·ness (ˈkīn(d)nəs) noun

The quality of being friendly, generous, and considerate

~ Google

See that no one repays another with evil for evil, but always seek after that which is good for one another and for all people.

~ Bible 1 Thessalonians 5:15 ESV

Compassion, as we saw in the last value, is an internal value. Therefore, the value of "kindness" can be explained as an external expression of the compassion that is in our heart. I believe that sportsmanship and kindness are interrelated with one another. You cannot have good sportsmanship without being kind to your opponent. Sportsmanship is "fair and generous behavior or treatment of others, especially in a sports contest" states Google. Kindness is a key part of fencing; we have to show kindness (good sportsmanship) all the time.

As we develop the value of kindness, in our lives, we will also increase friendships. Without a base of good friends, so many things in life can and will most likely be more difficult.

I know this all too well. While in elementary school, I did not have many friends. It wasn't from lack of trying. My family wasn't well off; you could say we were poor. We had food to eat and a place to live, but we didn't have all the extras. We never had brand name clothing. We bought clothes from low-end budget department stores, or my mom would make them. We never owned a new car and would do all the car maintenance repairs ourselves. I also had a speech problem and stuttered, along with reading issues. I have always been heavy set, so I was picked on a lot.

I know all too well our example of the playground bully at the beginning of the chapter. I was on the receiving end of that many times.

Then around the fifth grade, one classmate began to befriend me. His name was Steve. Steve would invite me to his house, and to church. I never felt anything but kindness and love from him, his family and his church. I could be myself around all of them. My status at school and home never changed. I still didn't have many friends. But, from that day forward, I looked at myself differently. Later after high school, I worked a retail job and we needed more help. I asked Steve to apply. We worked there for three years together. He helped me celebrate my wedding and I was there for his wedding as well. All because of one act of kindness (friendship and generosity), I now have a lifelong friend.

How lonely I felt before my encounter with Steve. At that time in my life, I didn't know if I would ever have good friends, let alone be loved. God made us to need others; God never wanted us to be alone.

In life, as in sports, you need others to help you to become better. Even major athletes who are exceptionally good at their sport need team members, trainers, coaches, family and most of all they need opponents. If we were able to go back in time and see these athletes growing up, we may see a life of sportsmanship (kindness) working in their lives and the same sportsmanship extended to them.

As you saw with my example of my lifelong friend Steve, it can be a simple action or deed like asking someone to church or to your house. Here are a few actions you can do to show kindness: being polite, giving, expressing appreciation, and being considerate.

**Being Polite**

Here are some basic things you can do to show politeness to others around you.

- Use words like “Please” and “Thank You”
- Respect adults, teachers and anyone in authority
- Do not interrupt when someone else is talking
- When you’re talking with someone, look them in the eye
- Do not play with your phone while in a conversation
- Never use fowl language (curse/swear)

**Giving**

There are many ways to give other than money, such as lend a helping hand or give your time. Help a neighbor with their lawn by raking their leaves. Help a student with a project or help carry some of their books. You can give time by reading to younger students, visiting senior citizens in a nursing home or volunteering for clean up or garden projects in your neighborhood or city. Help a parent around the house with tasks that might not already be assigned to you, like washing dishes or taking out the garbage. This is just a small list of example areas in which to give.

**Appreciation & Consideration**

Take the time to let others know you appreciate what they have done for you. If you really want to surprise your teacher, after class go up to them and politely thank them for giving their life to teach you. They will remember that the rest of the day, if not their lifetime.

You could write a note or make a card for a local police officer or fire fighter, thanking them for protecting you and your family.

Everyone likes appreciation, for the things they have done. Have you ever finished cleaning your room, chores or homework and announced to your family you are finished, looking for some appreciation? Sometimes appreciation comes and sometimes it doesn't. But remember, God is always there and He appreciates you. The Bible says that when we give of our lives to serve others for Him, God will say, "Well done, good and faithful servant!" Matthew 25:21 (NIV).

Before you can really appreciate someone, you have to know what he or she has finished/accomplished in their life and what it may have cost them. You have to give other people's actions, duties and deeds consideration. Let's practice this recounting by looking at what a teacher's day could look like.

Most people became teachers because they wanted to help students. They want to see children be and do their best. They go to college to get a degree spending from four to six years on schooling. After college, they get their first teaching job. Every night they have to study for the next days' subjects, grade all the assignments for that day and make sure they have everything prepared for the next day. In the morning, they greet their students and apply all the knowledge they reviewed the night before for each subject. Once the day is done, they too go home. But they don't get to just sit back with their family. No, they grade all the assignments from that day, study their subjects, and make their plans.

They give up family time, movie time, TV time and sometimes dinner, all for their students and classroom. This is only a small part of their duties and job. In understanding this, I hope you appreciate your teacher a little more.

Now that we've looked at everything a teacher gives up for us, take time and think about what a police officer, firefighter, doctor, nurse, parent and grandparent go through. If you want to understand what they had to overcome or accomplish, take time to engage in a conversation with them.

My friend once shared with me that her brother was always playing one particular game on his phone. As parents do, they were continually asking him to get off his phone so he could engage with other people. One day she asked him about the game. He just came alive and told her all about the game for an hour. She still doesn't know how to play the game or even the name of the game. Two things happened in that hour: her brother connected with a person and he felt appreciated and loved. All this because she was truly interested in something he enjoyed and really listened to him.

True kindness is doing for others without expecting anything in return or looking for a reward. You have to be careful not to use kindness for manipulation or selfishness. Do not go into any act of kindness thinking, "If I do that for them, then they will do this for me." This is not kindness!

**You are Challenged to A Duel!**

In the back of this book, there are a couple questions and a knightly value challenge.

# HUMILITY

hu·mil·i·ty ( (h)yo͞o'milədē) noun

> A modest or low view of one's own importance; humbleness.
>
> ~ Google

Do nothing out of selfish ambition or vain conceit. Rather, in humility value others above yourselves.

~ Bible Philippians 2:3 NIV

Children, obey your parents in the Lord: for this is right.

~ Bible Ephesians 6:1 NIV

Let me be clear about the definition from Google. It is not saying you are not important; God created you and has made you important. As you can see in the first Bible scripture, it is saying we should value others greater than we do ourselves.

We all like to be right; when we are right, it makes us feel good and feel significant. It also makes applying the value of humility in our life harder. Humility will cause us to admit things like, "I was wrong", "forgive me", "I made a mistake", or that we do not have all the right answers or correct actions.

We have to be able to admit our failures and mistakes; this can only help us to be more successful in life. The Bible states in Proverbs 28:13 (EVS) "Whoever conceals his transgressions will not prosper, but he who confesses and forsakes them will obtain mercy." In other versions of the Bible, the word "transgressions" in this verse translates to "mistakes".

While in my early thirties, I worked in the office of a newly formed construction company. I was their first full-time employee. I had many office skills that gave me the ability to do all types of varied duties the company needed. I learned how to draw site plans, schedule contractors and manage construction projects and contacts.

The company was growing fast. Within a year and a half, we brought two other employees into the office. One worked directly with contractors and took over as project manager including many of the duties that had been my responsibility. The other was a financial controller who took very little of my office duties. The owner asked if I could take on some additional duties and I accepted without knowing what all was involved.

It seemed that all the focus was on the two new employees and their duties. They received extra training and they sat in on various meetings. I felt as if I went from number one employee to number three. Within the next six months, I began sensing that the owners were not pleased with my level or quality of work.

I began to evaluate what I was or wasn't doing and if I should approach the owners. I determined that some of my work quality was lower than it should be and that I didn't have the right skill sets needed for the added duties. So, I made an appointment with the owners.

Days before the meeting I began to develop my argument about how "I did not have proper training", how "I was not included in all the meetings" and so on. I had all the points lined up in my head; I was ready for an argument. I was not clothed in humility, but felt I was prepared.

The meeting was not at the main office, but at one of the model homes, we built. As I drove over there, I was rehearsing my case to myself, but God was also listening. God showed me that I needed to be humble when talking to the owners. I decided to listen to God and throw out all of my arguments.

We sat down at the table and they requested I begin first since I asked for the meeting. I started by saying, "I believe I have over committed and over sold my abilities in taking on the additional duties and that they are lacking". I continued, "When you asked if I could take on the added duties, I did so without knowing what was going to be needed. This is on me and I understand I haven't done quality work for the company, the office or myself. I know that something needs to change." Both of them were looking at me, but not responding. I continued. "So if you need someone else who has the skill sets for these additional duties and would like me to resign, I'm requesting that I may have two weeks to find another job".

The room was silent for seemingly hours, but soon one of the owners spoke up. "We weren't expecting you to ask us to fire you; we thought you were going to ask for a raise." He told me that I was correct; they were not satisfied with my current work. They also told me they had all their arguments prepared about why they should not give me a raise.

You should always be confident when talking with your boss or employer, but never in pride. If I would have gone in with my arguments, all puffed up with pride, the meeting could have gone very differently. I might have lost my job right there. Because I came confidently, but humbly to discuss the situation and acknowledge I needed training for skills I didn't already have, my employer decided to keep me on and helped me get the training I needed.

When you are walking in humility, you will be happier with yourself and others and it will cause you to succeed. When you're walking in pride, it's all about you. There are many benefits of walking in humility. You will have peace in your life and with others and you will have favor with God and people.

I don't follow sports teams generally; but I do like to watch an NFL game occasionally. Most of the time after a play, you see teammates helping each other up. What I really like to see is an opponent helping their team member to their feet. This is another sign of humility, when you can value the efforts of another, even if they are opposing you.

It takes humility to be able to discuss topics with people of opposing values, politically, socially, economically and even spiritually; to be able to listen to their side without reacting, getting offended or frustrated. Everyone has his or her own opinions. Some ideas are based out of a completely incorrect concept and wrong perceptions or information. If we stop listening to them, we will never be able to help them. Friends of mine taught me this saying: "Do you want to be right or do you want relationship!"

What my friends were saying was, you may have an opposing opinion, and it may be right, but you can lose a friendship through an argument. This does not mean you have to agree with them or state their opinion is correct. You may have to just let them know that "We disagree, and for the sake of our friendship let's agree to disagree on the topic."

Some truths we have to just stand up for and not worry about a friendship. As an example, your friend wants to steal an item from a store. This is wrong and you shouldn't just go along because you don't want to lose your friendship. You must speak the truth that it is wrong, and walk away from that situation and the friendship if necessary. If your friend does take an item and you are there with him/her at the time, you will be in the same amount of trouble as he/she is. Do not allow false humility to make you into a doormat that others can walk on.

Along with humility, we should also think of honor. They are two sides of the same value. You cannot have honor without humility or have humility without honor. When you humble yourself to your parent, teacher, or boss, you are in turn honoring them. When you humble yourself in a sports game loss, you are honoring your opponent. This is one of the reasons we shake the hand of our opponent at the end of a fencing match.

**You are Challenged to A Duel!**

In the back of this book, there are a couple questions and a knightly value challenge.

# QUIET STRENGTH / GENTLENESS

qui·et (ˈkwīət) adjective

carried out discreetly, secretly, or with moderation

~ Google

Strength (streNG(k)TH) noun

the quality or state of being strong, in particular

~ Google

gen·tle·ness (ˈjen(t)lnəs) adjective

1. having a mild or kindly nature or character
2. soft or temperate; mild; moderate

~ Dictionary.com

A gentle answer turns away wrath, but a harsh word stirs up anger.

~ Bible Proverbs 15:1 NIV

When I think of gentleness, I think of a person who attended the church I attend. His name was Jerry. Jerry was a big man who stood about 6'8" if not taller. We affectionately called him a 'Gentle Giant'. He had so much strength in his physical body, but was so gentle. Jerry would engulf my wife with his hugs, but never held her too tight. This is an example of Quiet Strength.

Let's take some time and break down quiet strength. Quiet strength, I believe has two components: a quiet spirit and true power. The Bible says in First Peter 3:4 NIV "Rather, it should be that of your inner self, the unfading beauty of a gentle and quiet spirit, which is of great worth in God's sight." In addition, Proverbs 29:11 ESV "A fool gives full vent to his spirit, but a wise man quietly holds it back."

**Quiet Spirit**

A quiet spirit is meekness. Meekness is not weakness, it is power under control. To be in control, you need to be at peace with knowing that God is working through you and also knowing you aren't holding on to negative emotions or acting out of those negative emotions.

Have you ever entered the classroom and the teacher is having a bad day (not so quiet of spirit). It causes a heaviness in the room and no one seems to be able to move. Everything that is done seems to be wrong in her eyes. Even when your teacher asks about an assignment in a nice voice, the request seems to be so harsh.

The shyer students tend to feel all the pressure and say nothing, where the stronger willed students will push back. Everyone between the two points are also miserable. This is a very hard environment to get anything done. If you could, you would like to leave, but that isn't an option.

I have been in many work places that have the same situation. One person isn't at peace, so no one there is at peace. The world says this about families: "If mama's not happy, no one is happy" or "Happy wife, happy life". Even though these are ungodly beliefs, (we'll cover that in a later value) the pressure is the same, and the house is not at peace. This doesn't occur only with the mom or wife. The unrest can be generated by any family member, such as an over-worked father or a sibling battling depression or an addiction.

If any one of these hurting people would take a moment, collect their emotions (feelings) and deal with their own frustration, this would create a very different environment for all. We are unable to change or control other people; we can only change ourselves.

**Power / Strength**

Strength is not only physical, but can also be spiritual, economic, educational, or even relational (family). You can leverage every one of these areas, even against others. Strength obtained on our own merit alone is not true strength. True strength comes from God, and from searching to find Him. First Chronicles 16:11 ESV states "Seek the Lord and his strength; seek his presence continually!"

It's not a power struggle kind of strength, but a respectfully firm, quiet viewpoint, slow to respond inappropriately, and never too "self-important" to do the right things or the little things.

I have read that Navy Seals are consistently referred to as "quiet professionals". They are very skilled and extremely trained, but retain a modest attitude. They have the physical strength to overpower enemies, but the ability to restrain the same power when needed. They continually display the value of quiet strength.

I have volunteered in every church I have belonged to for years. When I was in my mid-twenties, I started to work on the church's soundboard. I had experience in selling and setting up soundboards when I worked for Radio Shack, but limited time actually running them. Two men at the church that had been doing it for years trained me. I have worked in the sound department at my local church and at other churches/conferences. I had a season where a leader was telling me how to set the controls on the soundboard. I knew that the information presented was not completely correct, but would not hurt the system, so I left the controls set as requested. I am a man under authority so I did what the leader asked.

I decided to walk in quiet strength; I had years of experience on the soundboard (strength), and wanted to apply a quiet spirit. Therefore, I ran the soundboard the way the leader requested for several months.

Over that time, I attempted to change some of the settings back, respectfully trying to explain to the leader why these settings would not always work correctly. The leader requested again that I keep it the way he believed it should be. I just answered him agreeably. Remembering the scripture above Proverbs 15:1 "A gentle answer turns away wrath, but harsh words stir up anger."

This continued until the church had a guest speaker/musician in for Sunday morning service. As we were setting up the guest's equipment, the leader noticed the setting, and we began our regular conversation. This time it ended differently because the guest speaker spoke up. He told the leader that I was correct and the soundboard does not work like that. I passed the test. I had walked out quiet strength.

Some of you might be thinking, "You should have said, 'I told you so!'", while pointing your finger in the leader's face. Or, "You could have ended it months earlier, if you would have loudly thrown around your years of experience of how you sold and set up sound systems."

Neither of the above options would have developed the value of "quiet strength" in my life. If I had forced my way by getting loud, this would have damaged or caused a valuable relationship with that leader to be lost. Our society has made it so easy to throw away relationships all under the premise of "I was right". As I mentioned earlier, "Do you want to be right, or have relationship".

When we walk in this value of quiet strength, it shows that we have passed the test, and succeeded, and that we do not need to show everyone our success. You do not have to be the loudest or most eye-catching person to have success, just have quiet strength and persistent forward motion toward God and your goals.

**You are Challenged to A Duel!**

In the back of this book, there are a couple of questions and a knightly value challenge.

## DISCIPLINE

dis·ci·pline (disəplən) noun

> The practice of training people to obey rules or a code of behavior ~ Google

For God has not given us a spirit of timidity, but of power and love and discipline.

~ Bible 2 Timothy 1:7 NASB

Set a guard, O LORD, over my mouth; Keep watch over the door of my lips.

~ Bible Psalm 141:3 ESV

Every athlete exercises self-control in all things. They do it to receive a perishable wreath, but we, an imperishable.

~ Bible 1 Corinthians 9:25 ESV

When most of us hear the word discipline, we think of punishment. Punishment is a penalty imposed for an offense; this is not typically the meaning for discipline. No one likes punishment but most people typically do not mind correction or discipline. We all like to have caring and loving people in our life who will give us guidance and correction. The Bible says that God disciplines the ones he loves. Jesus had a group of followers, called His disciples.

Google defines a disciple as "a follower or student of a teacher, leader, or philosopher". The difference between disciple and discipline is that a disciple is a person who is willing to be trained, educated and taught. To discipline is to train by instruction, practice or a code of conduct (values). A disciplined person is in fact a disciple.

From the above paragraphs, you can see that we need certain

things to have discipline:

1. A leader (instructor, teacher)
2. A follower (student)
3. A set of shared values. Why would you want an instructor who does not have the same values as yourself

I see three distinct areas of discipline:

1. Imposed
2. Self
3. True

These three areas can run independent from one another, but also in tandem. Let's look at these closer.

## *IMPOSED DISCIPLINE*

We have all been under imposed discipline. If you have ever been in public school, there is a teacher over you and your classroom. You learn many different disciplines through quizzes, assignments and homework, but you also learn time management by having to get up early and having pre-set schedules for classes, lunch, gym, and electives like music and art. You learn important social skills; how to work and play with others, problem resolution and how and when to speak up. These are but a few of the disciplines you learn in school.

We learn early in our school life that by submitting to these educational disciplines, we are able to advance along academically and in our friendships. We accept these imposed disciplines because our parents, grandparents and society teach us to.

As you advance within the educational system, you may

begin to think you have moved from imposed discipline to operating in self-discipline. You are keeping track of the daily schedule, participating in after-school activities while making sure you have time for homework. You may even have a part-time job. You learned and accomplished a lot, but you are still only operating in a fraction of self-discipline.

If you stopped doing your class assignments or homework you would quickly see that you are in an imposed discipline system. Within the imposed system, you are safe to apply self-discipline, without the fear of getting out of balance. The imposed system will not let you destroy your future by getting so far off track that you cannot recover. The imposed discipline system is not in itself evil or bad, it is just another training process.

The educational system is not the only aspect of imposed discipline in our current society. It is also found in our military, and even in the correctional system. Every one of these imposed discipline systems are designed to help you develop and/or re-develop, yourself.

In the past, our nation used to participate in the disgraceful practice of slavery, which was another form of an imposed discipline system. But it was of course evil because it was never designed to help people develop further or to ever give them a way out of bondage.

You can see imposed discipline within the Bible any time the Israelites were taken into captivity or occupied by another nation. The Hebrews lost their ability to make their own life choices. Even though they were in a form of slavery, the Israelites were still able to work on and develop their own self-discipline, which caught the eye of God.

## *SELF-DISCIPLINE*

Self-discipline is a set of values that keeps us from going the wrong way in life. Therefore, we set self-directed values to help us stay on our own path. We all have encountered people, who do not set any values, or ignore their values; they end-up in some very hard and difficult places. Your values are about what you do when no one is watching just as much as when someone is.

Self-discipline is all up to you. You were training for this all those years you were going through your elementary and secondary school years. While you were in the imposed discipline system, you were beginning to apply "self-discipline". Imposed and self-discipline are designed to work together.

I have seen high school students that seemingly do just enough to get a passing grade, putting in as little effort as possible on schoolwork and focusing more on friendships, popularity and athletic events.

Once they transition from high school to college and have to pay for their own college education, they step right into self-discipline. They apply all the disciplines they half-way applied in high school. They set personal values about what types of grades are acceptable, how much effort they are willing to invest and the time limits on athletic and social events.

You will always need to review, adapt and apply new self-disciplines. You may have to change some values because you may have set them higher than reasonably attainable. If you set a value of "my acceptable grades are all "A"s you may have to adjust it to something like: "I will give 100% effort in every course". If you get an "A" in every course, great but if you get a "C" but applied yourself 100%, you accomplished your value.

Once you move from college to the work world, you will also have to set new values and adjust other personal values. One of my life values is honesty. When I was in my mid-twenties, I began working at a bank on a college campus. I had to handle large amounts of cash every day. There were days that I would handle thousands and thousands of dollars.

Every fall, at the beginning of the college school year the bank would have a large number of international students opening accounts. Most of them were not fluent in English, and were difficult to understand.

One day an Asian student came to my window to make her opening deposit. She gave me $8,000.00 in hundred dollar bills. Her deposit slip was written out for $6,000.00. I tried to explain she gave me too much, but because of the language barrier, I was not getting this across to her. She did not want to change the deposit slip or take back the extra money.

A flitting thought ran through my head; I could just keep it and no one would know, but my value of honesty kept me from going down a wrong path.

I took all her money, made one deposit for $6,000.00 and gave her the receipt. Then I filled out another deposit slip for $2,000.00 and deposited that into her account. I tried to give her the other receipt, but she did not want it. I filed it with my daily paper work in case I needed it later.

As far as I know, the student did not come back and ask about the other $2,000.00. I thought perhaps a friend with less of a language barrier came to the bank and talked with another teller or office person and found the other deposit.

Your values will keep you from making choices that could cause future issues and heartaches. If I would have taken that students money and disregarded my values, it would have been easier to take the next person's money. Then that would not have been enough money and I would begin to create other ways to steal more money. When you disregard your values, it becomes a vicious cycle, making it harder and harder to return to them, similar to addictions.

This is where most of our addictions come in, through a lack of personal values applied to our lives. I am not talking about just drug or alcohol abuse. This can be in any area of our life. Even healthy things like exercise, if taken to an extreme can become unhealthy in your life and with others. If we decide to ignore our values, we are in jeopardy.

Simply put, self-discipline is a code of conduct (values) that will guide you through your life decisions. The enforcement of the code is not by another person, but internally by your conscience.

## *TRUE DISCIPLINE*

Sometimes it is easier to make excuses and tell our conscience that it is ok to do something against our values just this time. This is why the next step in discipline is so important; I call it "True Discipline". The only way to have true discipline in your life is by submitting to another person. This could be a teacher, boss, or a spiritual leader, and always God.

Unlike imposed discipline, with true discipline you have the option to choose the mentors you align with. I believe that it takes more than just one mentor in our lives to have balance. You give these mentors the right and privilege to help you develop the character values you desire in your life.

When you are looking for the right mentors, there are a few key items to look for. It should be someone who:

- Inspires you
- Has the desired character values working in their life
- Is open to being a mentor
- Has a relationship with Jesus Christ (very important but not always required)

Growing up, I had my dad, an older brother and two uncles in my life. My grandmother once asked me why my uncles treated me more like a son than a nephew. I kind of felt that way also, but didn't think anyone else noticed. As I thought through her question, I realized that they were like father figures because they were my mentors. My father was my mentor in employment values. When it came to providing financially for a family and developing a good work ethic, this was my father all the way. One of my uncles is an accomplished businessman. He sent me investment advice and advised me in my career choices. My other uncle embraces life to the fullest and is very artistic. He taught me to enjoy everything to the fullest and not to get caught up in materialistic traps. My brother is nine years older than I am. He displays an unconditional love to anyone he meets and he just loves people.

I was able to receive impartation in my life from all of these men. Not all of them had Jesus in their lives, but they had the character values I needed. Aside from my family, I had many more mentors. Most of them are in the kingdom of God. I have had input from many pastors and leaders. Some I had deeper relationships with than others, but I received from them all. I don't think I would be the person I am today without all the mentors I've had in my life. The greatest mentor I've ever allowed to have input into my life is the Holy Spirit.

Growing up, my family did not go to church much. When I was 22 years old, I gave my life to Jesus Christ and received the Holy Spirit. The Holy Spirit became the best mentor I've ever had. Christians are instructed to be like Christ. The Holy Spirit guides and helps us to accomplish that.

Even with all the earthly mentors I had, not one of them can compare to the Holy Spirit. The Holy Spirit goes everywhere I go and helps me keep my character values in my life. He has become an added strength to my conscience. I have a greater resolve to display not only my own character values, but also the character of Christ.

> "The Advocate, the Holy Spirit, whom the Father will send in my name, will teach you all things and will remind you of everything I have said to you."
> ~ Bible John 14:26 NIV

Once you accept Jesus Christ as your Lord and Savior, you will also receive the Holy Spirit, and He will be with you, leading you into all righteousness and truth. I have included a prayer in the worksheet in back.

**You are Challenged to A Duel!**

In the back of this book, there are a couple questions and a knightly value challenge.

# EVEN-TEMPERED

e·ven-tem·pered (ēvən'tempərd) adjective

Not easily annoyed or angered

~ Google

The one who has knowledge uses words with restraint and whoever has understanding is even-tempered.

~ Bible Proverbs 17:27 NIV

If you live alone on a deserted island, and this book just washed ashore, you probably have not been annoyed by someone else. For the rest of us, we live in a world where we all have family, classmates, neighbors and other relationships and can be annoyed or angered.

No matter what, people are going to be people. They are going to act in their own best interest. They are going to give you every opportunity to be irritated and annoyed.

Have you ever been walking down a hallway, on a sidewalk, or an aisle in a store, and someone is walking slower, taking up most of the walkway? You tried to get by them, and couldn't seem to catch a break. What is going through your mind? "What's wrong with you Bozo?", "Come on, really?" You are just slightly irritated, but if it keeps happening, you begin to get angry.

Getting irritated or angry is not wrong; what you do with that anger is the real issue.

> "In your anger do not sin": Do not let the sun go down while you are still angry, and do not give the devil a foothold.
>
> ~ Bible Ephesians 4:26-27 NIV

Keeping your temper when things are not going right can be difficult, but not impossible. Getting angry or annoyed takes a lot of physical strength. After an episode, you sometimes feel like you could sleep all day.

Growing up I had a short fuse on a very large powder keg of anger. All my life, it seemed to me that, I was picked on, disliked and rejected. This caused me to be able to take insults and razzing. My fuse was short but also wet; it took a lot for my fuse to be lit. But once it was lit, it burned fast. Watch out, it's going to blow!

One evening I was with my girlfriend (now wife); we accepted an invitation to her friend's house for a party. She was a senior in high school and it was going to be a holiday party. We had gone to many of her friend's parties in the past. They were typically quiet with no drinking; we would just have great times.

This night was different; her friend did not tell us that her parents were not going to be home. She also had invited other friends who we were not familiar with. Upon arriving, the first thing we noticed was some people were openly drinking.

Still living out of my rejection, I began to see how the other boys were judging us. Then the taunting and joking began for about an hour; derogatory comments and name calling. She was doing better than I was with the comments. She didn't have the victim mentality that I did. I wanted to protect her, not just from the taunting, but also from seeing the ugly part of me; my anger that I had been hiding.

I told her that we needed to leave. Not affected by the

taunting and joking, she wanted to stand against this bullying. I asked her again to leave and she refused and just stared back at them. One of the so-called gentlemen, made a disrespectful comment about her.

I could smell the scent of sulfur in the air; the match was lit, and it just touched my short fuse. In seconds I burst into a flame of rage. I turned toward the door that was at the back of the house. On my way to the back door, I hit the wall with my fist. I just wanted to get to my car to let this fire of my ugly rage burn out.

Another longtime friend of my wife, who was also at the party, came out to check on me. She allowed me to vent without any judgement. If you knew my wife's friend at the time, you'd agree that was amazing. She threw a wet blanket of love over my fire mess, smothering the rage. I wish I would have had Jesus in my life at that time, but she showed me my first glimpse of Jesus; an acceptance and unconditional love I always wanted. That night was the first time we really became friends too.

Once the fire was out, I was so tired. I just wanted to go home and sleep. So, I went back into the house to get my wife. As the door opened, and I walked back into the room, a deafening silence came over the entire house. Everyone stopped and just stared at me as I walked over to my wife, took her by the hand, and led her out of the house. As I was walking out, I saw the hole I made through the plaster and wooden lattice that made up the wall.

The next day I returned to the house to apologize for my actions. There were messes all over the house, evidencing how out-of-hand the party got after we left. My wife's friend accepted my apology and asked if I could fix the hole before her mother returned home. I was able to patch the hole and match the paint so that no one, not even her mom, would know what happened.

After that night, I wanted more of the unconditional love I had experienced and began seeking to find what I now know to be Jesus as Lord of my life. About a year after that dreadful night, I allowed the unconditional love and acceptance of Jesus into my life. Jesus removed my short powder keg fuse. He gave me a very long fuse, wrapped in the wax of his unconditional love and acceptance, that I could instead be a candle to give His light to others who need Him.

About three years later, my wife and I married. We were able to invite our friend and her husband to church with us. They came to know Jesus as I did. We served in the same church for many years.

When you get angry, you have to be careful not to act or react out of your feelings. You need to recognize and deal with your feelings.

In my life experience above, I could have been angry for so many reasons. I could have been angry with my wife's friend who hosted the party, the so-called gentleman, the drinking, etc. To break down my feelings in simple terms "I FELT angry ABOUT the crude comments BECAUSE I thought I was rejected and unloved." My anger stemmed from a lack of acceptance, not from the people at the party. Through Jesus Christ, I now know I am accepted and loved.

To get a hold on my feelings as I did above, I used a tool called the Feeling Formula. Ministry friends of ours, Dave and Linda from Paraklesis Ministries introduced this tool to us. My wife and I have been using it for years and it's one of the tools we teach anyone who will listen.

It works like this:
Fill in the blanks to this simple statement. There are a couple guidelines to follow to make it work which are listed below.

I FEEL ______________________________
ABOUT ______________________________
BECAUSE ______________________________

Guidelines for "I FEEL"

- Use only emotional description words
- Do not use LIKE such as "I Feel Like…"

Rules for "ABOUT"

- Do not use a person's name. If that person never changes, you will never be able to resolve your feelings.

Rules for "BECAUSE"

- Start by using the phrase "I think" or "I am".
- This could bring up other feeling words that you might have to work through in another Feeling Formula.

Once you have the "BECAUSE" this is typically what we call an ungodly belief – something we believe that is not true or not completely true. We usually didn't realize it. We then replace that ungodly belief with what God is saying about us, a Godly belief. Take this ungodly belief to God in prayer and ask Him what He says about you.

In my life example, I said, "I FEEL angry ABOUT the crude comments BECAUSE I think I am rejected and unloved."

After finding these ungodly beliefs, I decided to do one at a time, first "Rejection". I prayed that God would show me how He saw me. I heard in my mind that "I am accepted by Jesus" and "I am a Child of God". These would become my new Godly beliefs.

Again, I prayed about being "Unloved". Again I heard in my mind that "God loved me so much, that He gave His Son for me", my new Godly belief.

"I am accepted" replaced "Rejected" and "God's Love" replaced "Unloved". I then searched the Bible, found scriptures that confirmed these new Godly beliefs and began to recite the Godly beliefs and scripture for the next 21 days.

We can't change other people. We can't change how they treat others or what happened in the past. The only thing we can change is ourselves. Once you can really see why you're angry, you can obtain healing through the Holy Spirit.

This is why the scripture Ephesians 4:26-27 NIV continues with, "Do not let the sun go down while you are still angry and do not give the devil a foothold."

By dealing with our feelings quickly, we will not hold grudges against friends, family or others. If we allow these feelings to continue, anger can turn into criticism and self-hatred. Unchecked, it progresses to feelings of revenge until rage consumes you. Any one of these stages of the anger progression can cause you to react wrongly (sin), even to the point of hurting someone else. The Bible warns us about this type of foothold.

Submit your feelings and your character values to the Holy

Spirit to see how to act or react in every situation. In the Bible it says "But everything should be done in a fitting and orderly way." I Corinthians 14:40 NIV. Our actions should always show the heart of God.

**You are Challenged to A Duel!**

In the back of this book, there are a couple questions and a knightly value challenge.

# CONTENT

con·tent (kən'tent) adjective

In a state of peaceful happiness - A state of satisfaction

~ Google

But godliness with contentment is great gain. For we brought nothing into the world, and we can take nothing out of it.

~ Bible 1 Timothy 6:6-7 NIV

Our foundational scripture Colossians 3:12-14 MESSSAGE Bible says "**content** with second place". It is hard when you get second place in today's world. Today's society sometimes teaches us that second place is a bad thing. It is not. To be CONTENT with second place shows true character.

To walk in the value of being content, you have to be comfortable and happy with who you are and how God made you. If you strive to fit into another person's mold, allowing that mold to define you, it will only produce frustration. This frustration can also come from a false perception of what you believe others expect of you.

Have you ever tried to live under someone else's seemingly unrealistic rules and never seemed to get the rules right, no matter how hard you tried?

Unfortunately, sometimes mentors, churches, businesses and our legal system (institutions) seem to do this. They create rules or laws out of good intentions, but not representative of the people they are working with. These above listed institutions should create any rules or laws based on the needs of the mentee and/or the majority of the community they service.

Everything we do is a choice. We choose where we live (city, state, nation) so we should obey those laws. When we choose a mentor, we should also listen and adhere to the rules or guidelines of that relationship. The same applies where you choose to attend church or work. The rules an institution develops is based on the foundation of their vision and mission statement, and in most cases should be using the Bible, or God's heart intentions.

Contentment is not a passive activity. We need to give 100% to whatever we are engaged in. By giving everything, we will know that we have done everything we can to succeed. If the project or organization fails, we will still be content with our efforts.

All the way though first grade to twelfth grade I struggled with school. I had a very hard time spelling and sounding out words and reading was painful. I always wanted to do well and I tried my hardest. I also struggled with speech difficulties. Inevitably, twice a year, the day I dreaded came: report card day.

My teacher would hand out the report cards. We had to take them home for our parents to see and sign. I would sometimes open the envelope first just to see how much trouble I was in. Or, I would intentionally forget and leave it in my desk. I once tried to tell my parents that we didn't get them yet. That didn't work well because I had two sisters in school with me.

I would eventually hand over the report card and the same conversation would begin: They knew that I was smart, that I needed to focus, and that I needed to finish my homework. I never had a great report card. I would have settled for a good report card, but it never came.

My parents helped me through my speech difficulties; they had the school put me in speech therapy. I did not want to go into another therapy group for reading, which would only give the bullies more ammunition to pick on me. Therefore, I never told my parents about my reading problems. I would give 100% effort to every assignment and test. I became content with my grade knowing that I gave it my all.

Some might say I became apathetic about my grades, but I had interest, and concern. This is why I never stopped doing my best or quit school. So when my daughter began school, I never pressured her for "A"s I would tell her that if she gave 100% effort toward the class and got "C"s or even "D"s I would be ok with that.

Throughout her school years I held to my view of 100% effort is all I was looking for. She would bring home report cards of "A"s and "B"s. She wasn't content with that because they were not all "A"s. I had to explain many times that "B"s were ok because she gave 100%. After a while, she became content knowing she was putting in 100% effort and not as much emphasis was placed on the letter grade.

Being content is not just doing enough to get by or doing the "Status Quo". That is apathy: the lack of interest, enthusiasm or concern. If my daughter would have come home with a "D" in a subject, and we both knew she didn't try her hardest, there could have been punishment. This never happened though.

There is a story in the Bible about a master who gives his servants some money to watch over while the he is gone. When the master comes back, he wants an account from the servants. One servant had five bags of gold, invested it, and made another five bags.

> "His master replied, 'Well done, good and faithful servant! You have been faithful with a few things; I will put you in charge of many things. Come and share your master's happiness!'
>
> ~Bible Matthew 25:21 NIV

When we accomplish any task, we all would love to hear "Well done", from our parents, teachers and/or mentors. We all strive to receive praise and feel rejected if we do not. But, we don't have to if we are content with our own skills and performance, then that praise is an addition.

We have to choose to be content. There is not a list to reference or something we accomplish. Contentment is a heart issue. Loving yourself is a big start. Be nice to you, you are the only you, you have!

**You are Challenged to A Duel!**

In the back of this book, there are a couple questions and a knightly value challenge.

## FORGIVE

For-give (fər'giv) verb

Stop feeling angry or resentful toward (someone) for an offense, flaw, or mistake ~ Google

For if you forgive other people when they sin against you, your heavenly Father will also forgive you.

~ Bible Matthew 6:14 NIV

And when you stand praying, if you hold anything against anyone, forgive them, so that your Father in heaven may forgive you your sins."

~ Bible Mark 11:25 NIV

Walking out this value can be hard. When we are hurt, put-down, lied to, or even worse, feel that someone owes us and needs to pay.

When there is a major offense that is illegal, the perpetrator does need to pay according to our social and justice system. This is right, but we still need to walk in forgiveness towards them. This is definitely one of the hardest things to do.

With both minor and major offenses, we want our offender to be put in a mental jail and held there until we feel better. The problem is that we do not feel better, and they keep going as if nothing has happened. We are really the one behind bars; trapped by our own unforgiveness. We are unable to progress with our life, stuck there unable to get past that offense. We have the universal key: "forgiveness". It is right in our hand, to open our own jail and set us free.

God says in Deuteronomy 32:35 (NIV) "It is mine to avenge;

I will repay. In due time their foot will slip; their day of disaster is near and their doom rushes upon them."

We are taking the place of God by executing our own justice on an offender. God will not punish an offender if another person is doing it for Him. When we let the person go by extending "Forgiveness", then God can take over and execute the correct punishment. We do not know the heart of a person, but God does.

We may never see the full punishment or ever get an apology from the offender. We need to be content with letting God do His part. Most often, the offender does not even know what he or she did that was wrong.

It is never too late to extend forgiveness. As I have shared in the previous values, I had problems reading in elementary school. When I was in the fourth or fifth grade, I went to the library for a reading class.

I couldn't tell you what book I was trying to read, but I was unable to pronounce a word. The teacher had me go through every letter and make that letter sound. This worked sometimes, but not this day. I was stuck on this word; I just could not get the sounds to flow together. The teacher had other kids he had to work with, so he sat me in a cubical with the word written on a piece of paper.

I sat there for hours coming out every so often to try to pronounce the word to the teacher, with no success. The teacher even had me have my lunch in the same cubical. I began to blame myself and thought it was my fault and that I didn't deserve to have my lunchtime recess. When it came to the end of the day and all the other students had left for home on the school buses, the teacher finally told me the word was "ENOUGH" and proceeded to drive me home.

I can't remember ever seeing that teacher again. I don't know what happened. I know my reading did get better, so I could stop going to reading classes. He may have been a substitute teacher or just filling in for a short time. Perhaps my mother called about why I didn't come home on the bus. I don't know what happened.

I vowed in my heart that this would not happen again. So I decided I would not tell anyone that I was having a problem reading. I stopped reading anything I didn't have to. I didn't like or trust any teachers.

I allowed that hurt to turn into unforgiveness. I made my own judgement about that teacher and thought I was locking him up in a cell. What happened was the cell door locked and I was the one trapped behind bars. The teacher still had a job and lived his life as if nothing happened.

A couple years after I graduated high school, I went to a testing center and had my reading tested. I was at a fifth grade reading level. I was still locked in the cell I made with my judgement and my reading hadn't ever moved further than the fifth grade.

I began to work on my reading. I began telling myself "I can do all things through Christ who strengthens me". Other friends told me "Do not call yourself stupid anymore. You have the mind of Christ". I had my Godly beliefs even before I knew I needed them.

However, it wasn't until I learned how to use the Feeling Formula that I got full release from the jail cell of my judgement. I was able to forgive the teacher and my life changed.

Forgiveness is not forgetting. I still remember the details, but none of the hurts or judgements. Forgiveness is releasing others of offensive behavior, flaws, and mistakes so that you can live and love again.

This is not a one time and done process. You may have to go through forgiveness daily for a while. I began to forgive my teacher in my mid-twenties and had a total release in my early forties. We have to continually forgive until the full release comes.

If I would not have forgiven my reading teacher, I may not have written this book. I may not have ever gotten my two positions in a public school instructing fencing students and working in the IT department. I would have been trapped in my offense back in the fifth grade.

**You are Challenged to A Duel!**

In the back of this book, there are a couple questions and a knightly value challenge.

Developing knightly or Godly character values in our lives is a journey, not a destination. Therefore, you won't be surprised to find out that it is a continuous lifelong journey with many points to develop along the way. This may have been your first point or one of many.

Wherever you are on your journey through this study, I hope you have been allowing **Compassion** and **Kindness** to work in your life through **Humility** and **Quiet Strength.** I also hope you have applied **Discipline** in your life through the Lordship of Jesus Christ and the leading of the Holy Spirit along with some help from one or more good personal mentors. In addition, continue to be **Even-tempered** and **Content** in all things, walking out **Forgiveness**.

All of these are values developed internally with an external expression, which will affect others' lives. By using your newly obtained and applied values, you are becoming a community builder and world changer.

**GO OUT AND CHANGE YOUR WORLD!**

# FENCING FOUNDATIONS & SKILLS

# SAFETY

There are some basic safety protocols that as a class, we must follow for the safety of all.

Check your equipment prior to getting on the strip:

Foils, Epees, and Sabers Checklist:

1. Check the tip for wear and tear
2. Shake equipment by grip and if you hear a rattle sound, do not use; see an instructor
3. Look over the blade for proper bend
    - Foil: a single sloping bend toward the floor
    - Epee: a slight bend toward the floor
    - Saber: a slight bend to the right or left
4. Look to ensure no excessive rust or metal burrs
5. Always keep the equipment pointing toward the floor when not on the strip (Tips on Toes)
6. Never practice or swing equipment at anyone without all proper safety gear on both fencers
7. If you need two hands to put on your mask, lay your blade down first

Mask Checklist:

- Bib in good condition with no rips, tears, or fraying
- Mesh has no divots or dents and minimum rust

Jacket Checklist:

- In good condition with no rips, tears, or fraying
- Make sure the strap latches

Safety Tips:

- Wear good athletic clothing (gym shoes, lightweight shirt, gym clothes)
- Proper safety gear in good condition (minimum: mask and jacket)
- Make sure your opponent is also safe

- Never lose your temper
- Obey the Referee (President)
- Don't start fencing until referee says "Fence" and stop when he/she says "Halt"
- If you are sparring without a Referee, make sure you're both ready before starting
- Never turn your back on your opponent. Remember there are gaps in the back of your mask and collar which are not protected
- Do not run into your opponent or jostle him/her. Body contact and/or "Barging" is not allowed
- Keep your non-foil hand out of the way
- Holding the bib of your mask or bringing your hand in front of the target area is not allowed. It's also extremely painful to be hit on unprotected fingers
- Learn to make the hits firm, but with a **light touch.** You're not trying to run your opponent through

# PARTS OF THE FOIL

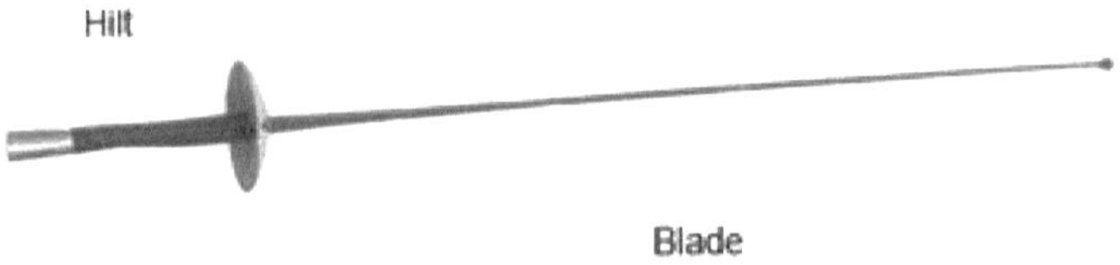


As with most swords, the foil is broken down into two major parts called the "Hilt" and the "Blade". The hilt is the lower portion of the sword, and the blade is the longer portion extending from the hilt. About one-fourth of the foil is the hilt and the blade makes up the remaining three-fourths.

## *THE HILT*

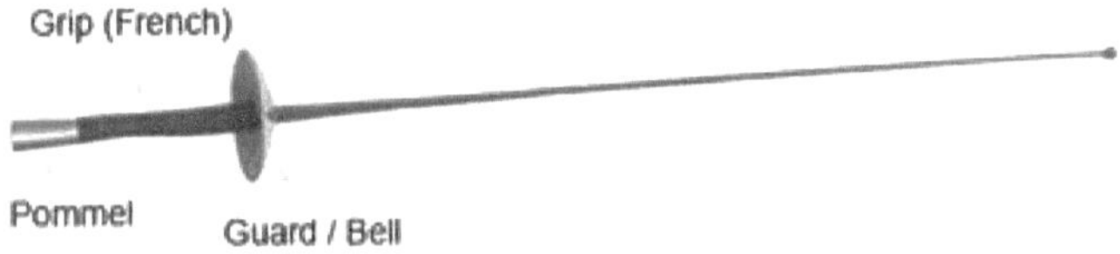


There are basically three parts to the Foil Hilt: the "Pommel", "Guard/Bell" and "Grip".

- The Pommel is the weighted end of the hilt and functions as the nut that holds the foil together
- The Guard is 9.5 to 12 cm in diameter and is positioned between the blade and the grip
- The Guard is designed primarily as a leverage point for executing parries and it also protects your hand during a bout
- The style of foil grip most often used in class is the "French" grip; it's a long, mostly straight, grip slightly formed to the hand for comfort

There are many other styles that are used throughout the world and most are designed to have the most ergonomic shape possible. These "Ergonomic Grips" are often referred to as "Pistol" Grips" as seen to the right.

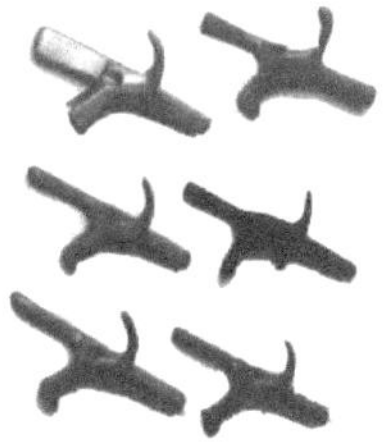

## *THE BLADE*

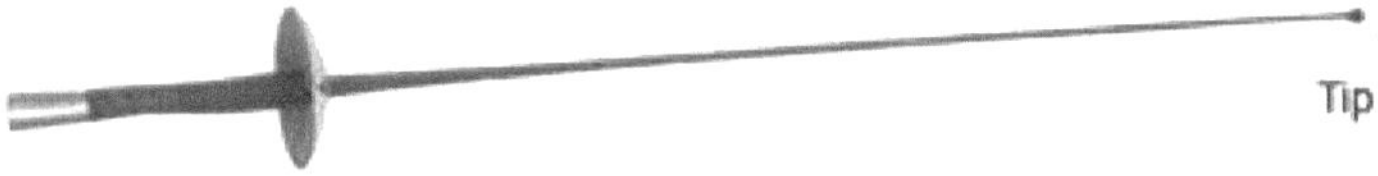


The three parts of the Blade that we cover in class are the Forte (fôr tā), Foible (foibəl) and Tip/Point.

- The forte is the strong part of blade where you do most of your defensive blade work in the parries
- The foible is in turn the weaker (though faster) part of the blade
- The Tip or Point is the area of the blade used to score touches; you must "set" the point of the blade to score a "touche" (touch) in Foil and Epee

Historically the tip of the blade was covered with cork and then the end was charred with a flame. This would cause an ash ring to show up on the white jackets, making it easier to determine whether the "touche" was scored. In modern electric tournaments, the tip is replaced by a push button. Once the touche is scored, the button completes a circuit to show who scored the touch. We use a slightly modified method to judge bouts in the classes. The Judges (Presidents) will keep an eye on both competitors to see who has right-of-way and who scored the touch, just as was done in the "Classical" period of fencing (No corks or flames are required).

## *FOIL, EPEE, AND SABER*

All three of the Olympic swords have the same structure and terminology. They all have different functionality and rules about how they score touches. Both the Foil and Epee may have either "French" or "Pistol" grips. The Saber has a large swooping guard to cover and protect the weapon hand and connect to the pommel.

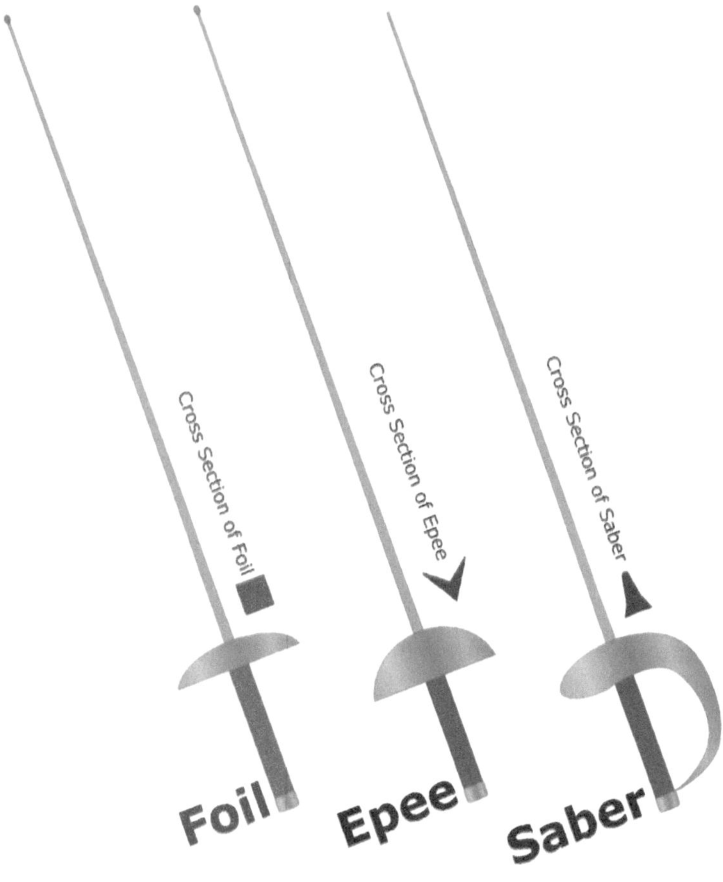

# EN GARDE / ADVANCE / RETREAT

## *EN GARDE*

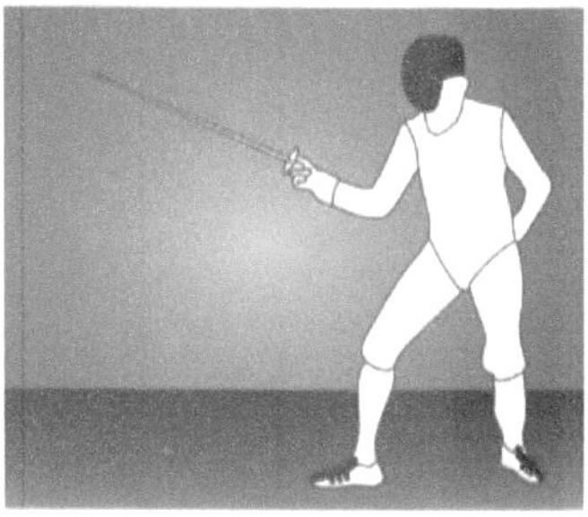

There are two basic positions in fencing. The first position is the En Garde. To get into a proper En Garde, you need your feet perpendicular to each other. Your feet should make an "L" shape, with the front foot pointed toward your opponent. Your heels should be shoulder width apart, with both knees bent, making sure the knees are directly over your heels. Your torso should be perpendicular to the back foot, keeping your shoulders directly over your hips, with your spine straight. You should look over your lead shoulder without turning your torso. Your back hand needs to be kept behind your torso, either on the back hip below the jacket or behind the back of your head. Your weapon arm holds the foil with the tip pointed toward your adversary's eyes. The bell guard should be at sternum level with your elbow about 5 to 6 inches in front of the torso.

## *ADVANCE*

How to execute an Advance step-by-step:

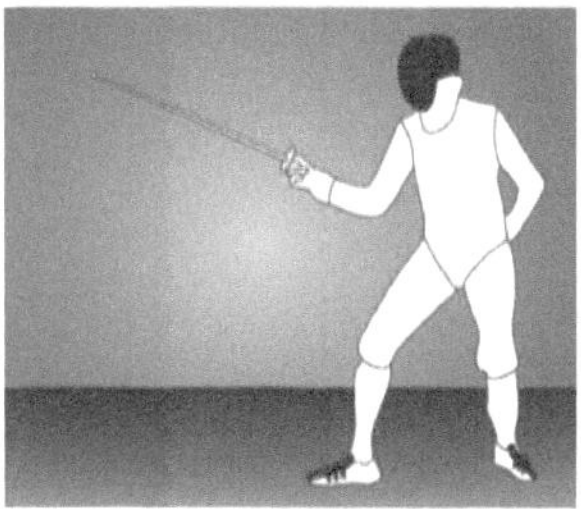

Start in the standard En Garde position

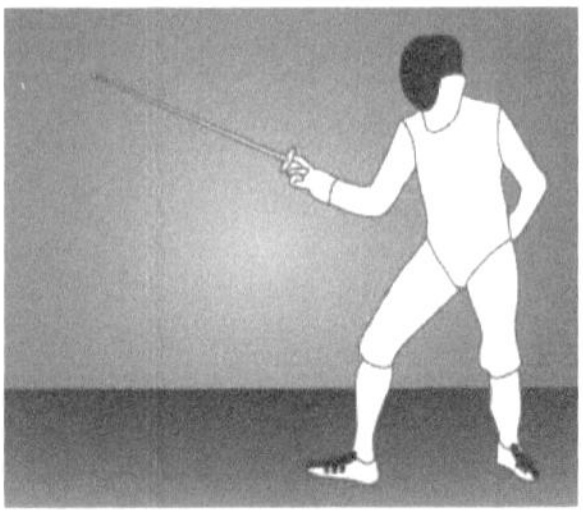

Raise the toes of the lead (front) foot

Slightly pick up lead foot

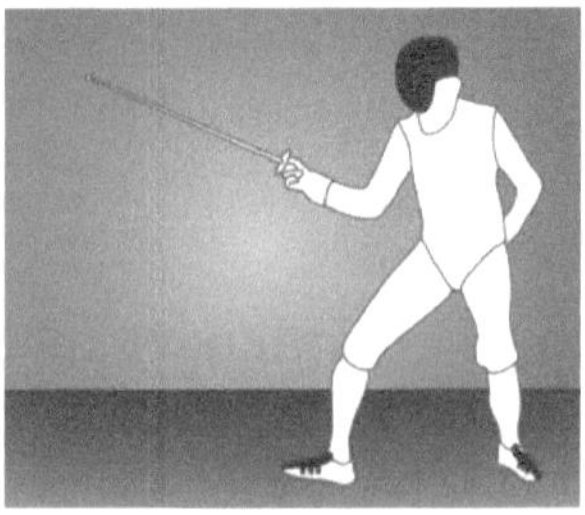

Push with back
leg causing your front foot to go forward

Place your heel first about 6" to 10" forward

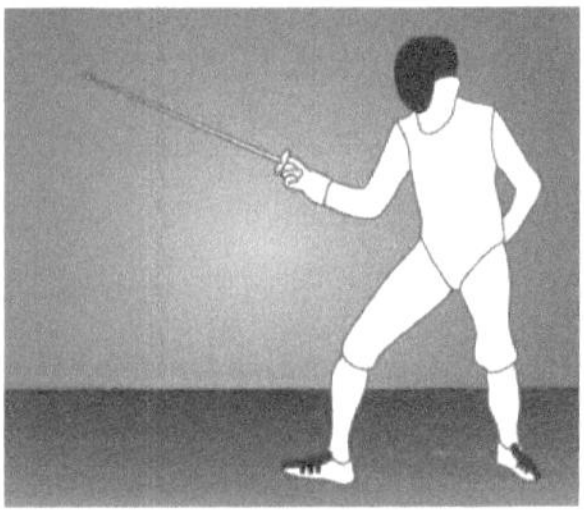

Follow with the back foot moving the same 6" to 10"

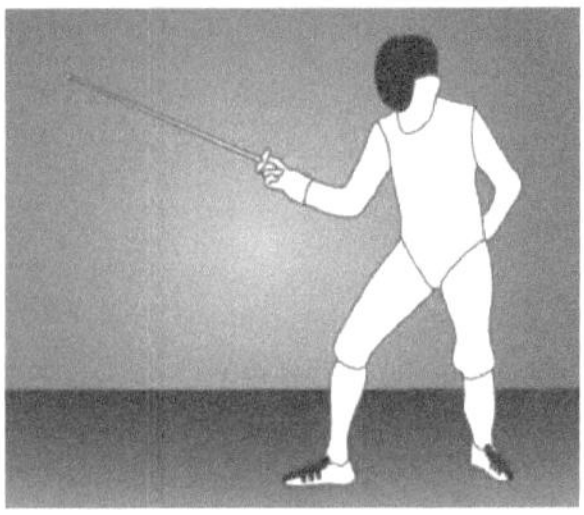

Return to the En Garde

## *RETREAT*

How to execute a Retreat step-by-step

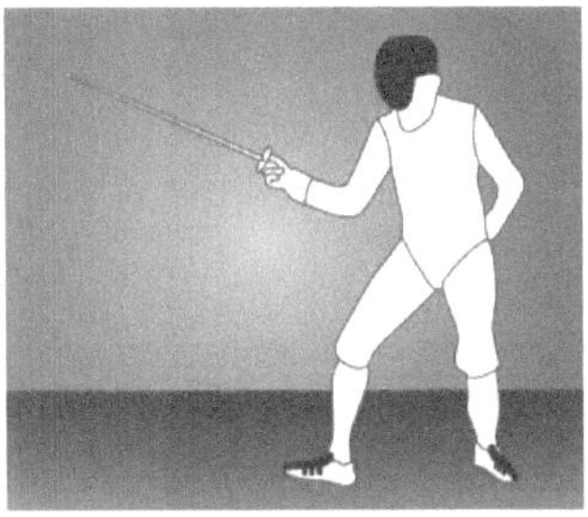

Starting from the
En Garde

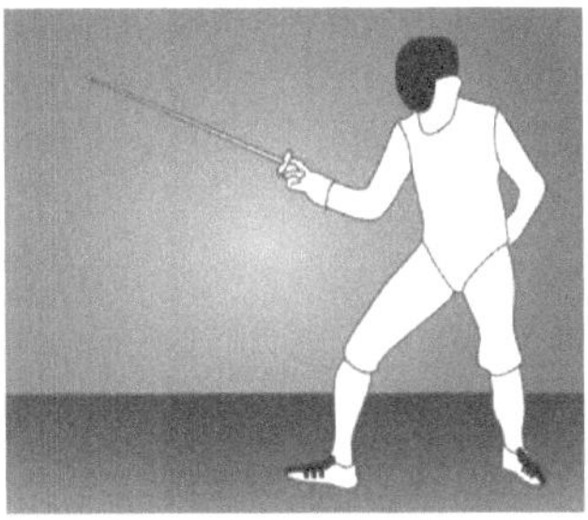

Move the back foot first
only 6" to 10"

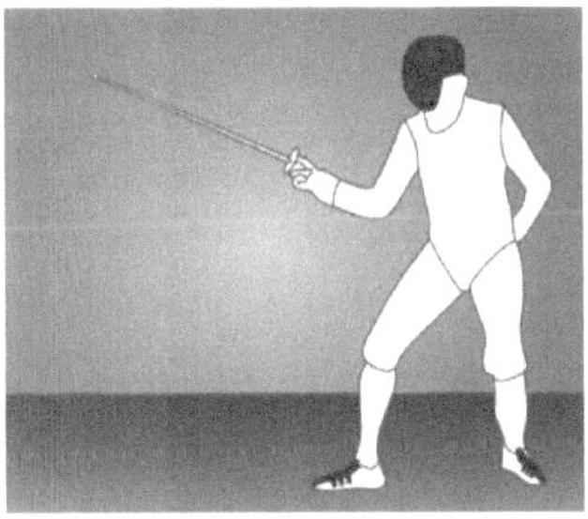

Follow with the front foot

# LUNGE / RECOVER

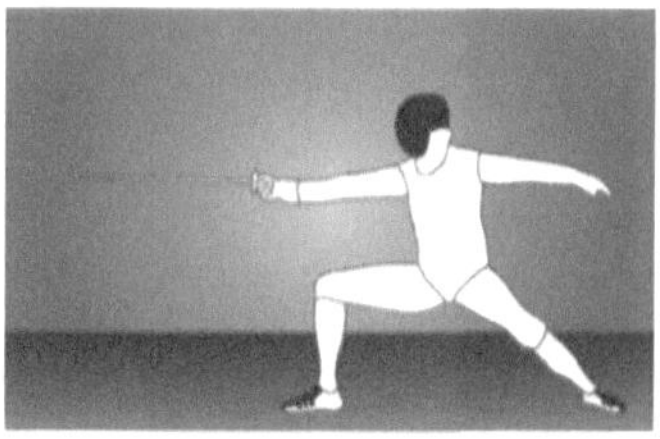

The "Lunge" is also known as the "Second Position". It's the primary offensive attack used in fencing.

There are variations:

- Lunge - moving the front foot to the maximum distance while still allowing you to recover
- Short Lunge - moving the front foot a minimum distance forward
- Low Lunge - same as the Lunge, but also extending your torso so it's directly over the front thigh
- Step Back Lunge - your weapon hand moves slightly forward as you step backward with your back foot leading, and drop into a lunge

Each of the lunges listed are used as different attacks, depending on the previous defensive or offensive moves your opponent has just made

- Lunge - you are attacking first, and your opponent is still in their En Garde position
- Short Lunge - your opponent has just moved in closer, but has not yet attacked
- Low Lunge - your opponent attacked on the high line, and you can safely drop under their attack to counter
- Step Back Lunge - You will not have right-of-way using this lunge, but utilize it if your opponent's attack falls short and you have a longer reach

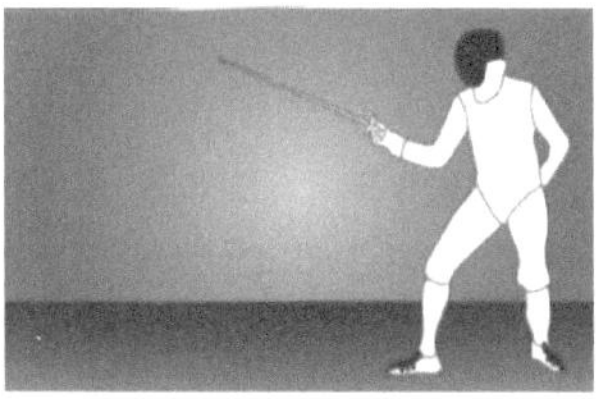

Start from En Garde

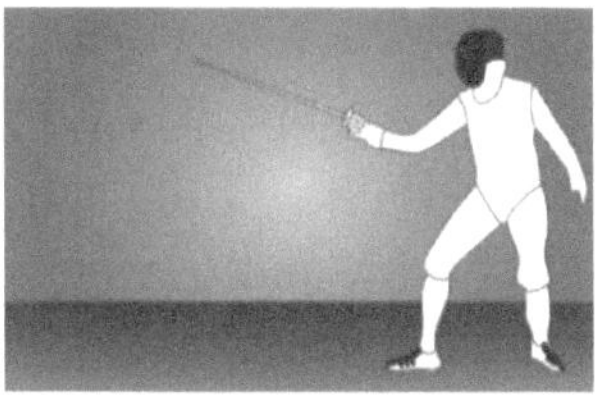

Begin by extending both arms while lifting your left foot

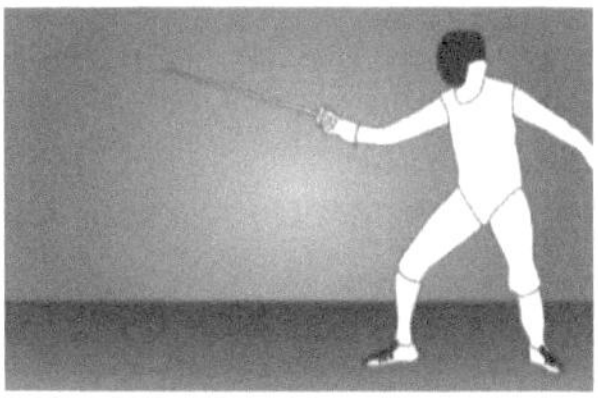

Lift the front foot while pushing off with your back foot

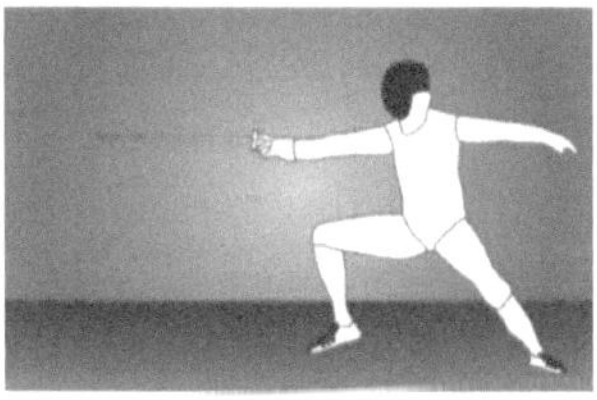

Straighten the back leg while leaving the back foot planted

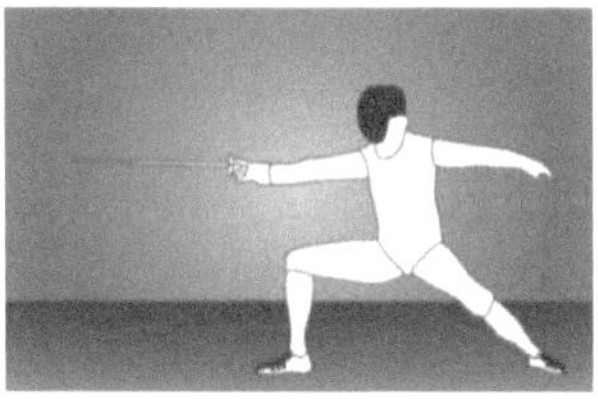

Land your front foot as the point of your weapon sets on your opponent

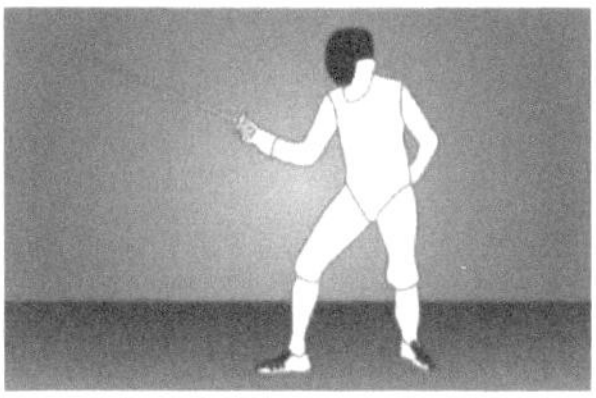

Recover back or forward as needed

## TARGET AREAS

Target Area is the area of the body that you are able to score touches on during a bout/match. The type of weapon you are fencing with will determine what the Target Area will be.

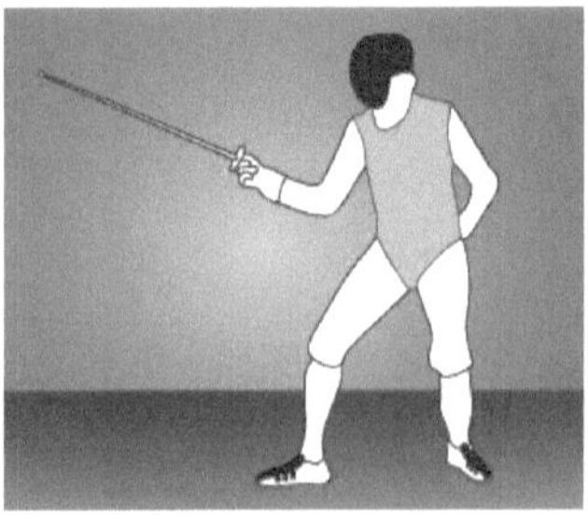

**Foil Target Area**

The Foil Target Area is comprised of the full torso (front and back), and the groin. The bib, mask, legs, and arms are invalid target areas. If the point lands under the bib and sets on the jacket, this is considered a valid touch. Modern rules have added the lower portion of the bib as valid target area.

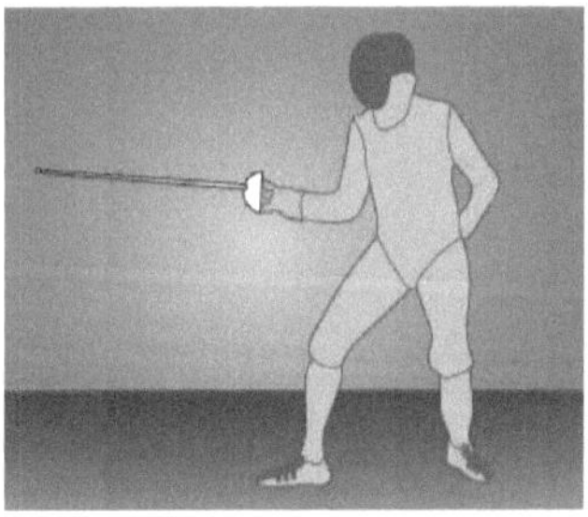

**Epee Target Area**

The Epee Target Area is comprised of the entire body from the top of the mask to the tip of the toes.

The only non-target area is the bell guard. Priority/Right-of-Way is NOT used in Epee.

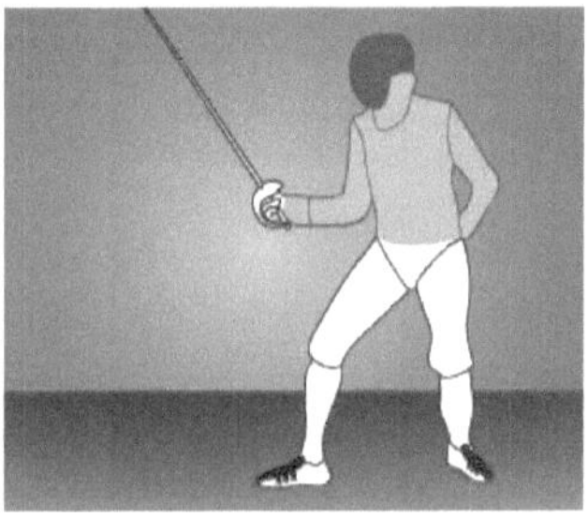

**Saber Target Area**

The Saber Target Area is comprised of everything above the waist, excluding the hands and the back of the head.

Priority/Right-of-Way is used in Saber.

## *"RIGHT-OF-WAY" OR PRIORITY*

Priority or "Right-of-Way" is used in Foil and Saber fencing to determine which fencer receives the point. Foil and Saber are conventional weapons.

> con·ven·tion - kən'ven(t)SH(ə)n/ noun
> a way in which something is usually done, especially within a particular area or activity
> ~ Google

Conventional weapons are governed by a set of rules and "priority" is one rule in both Foil and Saber. Generally, priority is determined by which fencer begins their attack first. In order to begin an attack, a fencer must threaten the target area of the opponent with the weapon. When doing a compound attack, the fencer must keep from withdrawing the weapon arm by bending the elbow.

The fencer who attacks first would maintain priority if:

- The opponent attacks into your attack
- The opponent attempts to avoid the touch, but fails to do so
- The opponent parries the attack, but pauses before the riposte (see glossary of terms)

The hit made by the opponent would have priority if:

- The opponent already has point-in-line
- The attacker makes a pause or withdraws the weapon arm during which time the opponent lands a touch
- The attacker does a compound attack and the opponent executes a touch which is in between the two attacks
- The opponent parries the attack and makes an immediate riposte

## INSIDE / OUTSIDE LINE

To determine which line the attack is coming from, you must first know the difference between the "Inside", "Outside", "High" and "Low" Lines.

**Inside / Outside line**

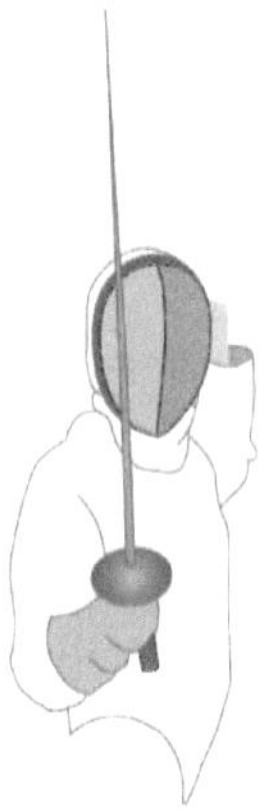

From the En Garde



An imaginary vertical line from the center of the bell

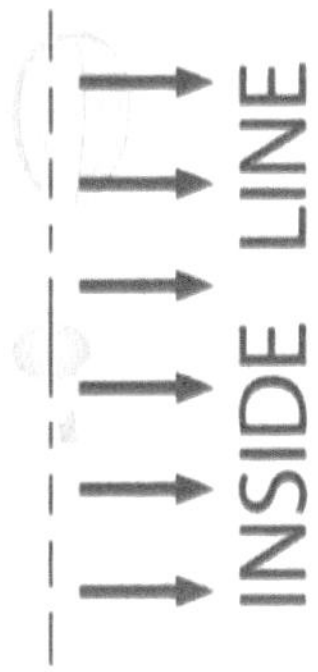


Everything to your front is your INSIDE Line

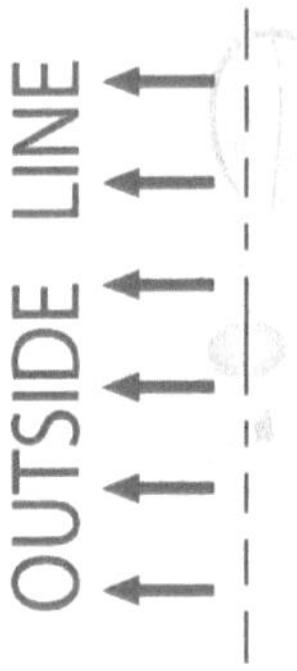


Everything towards your back is your OUTSIDE Line

**High / Low Line**

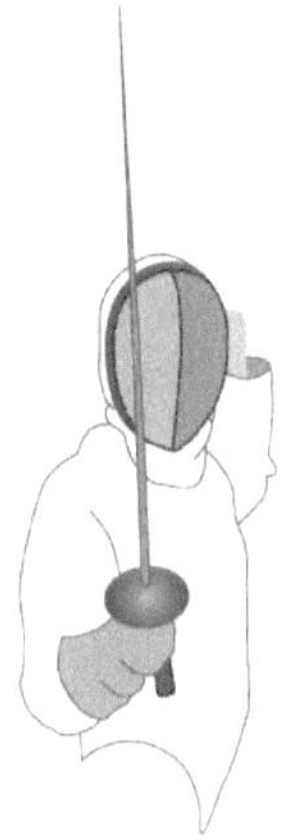

From the En Garde



An imaginary horizontal line
from the center of the bell

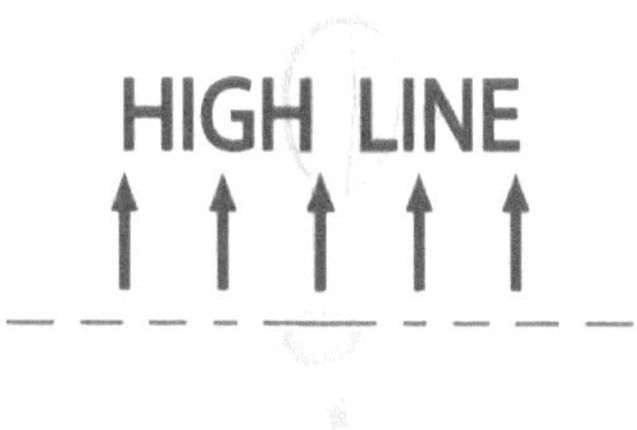


Everything above the bell
is your HIGH Line

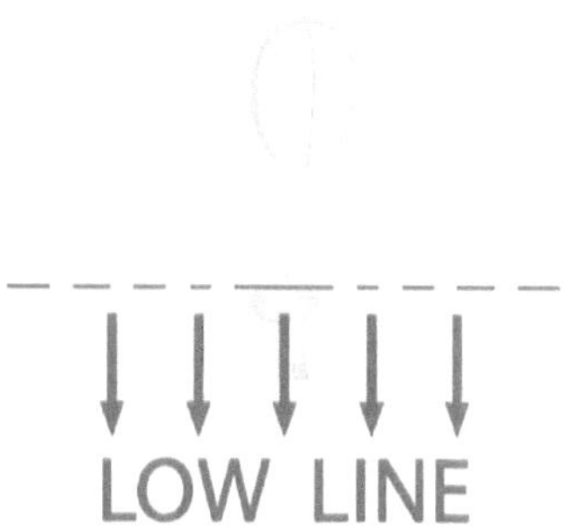


Everything below the bell
is your LOW Line

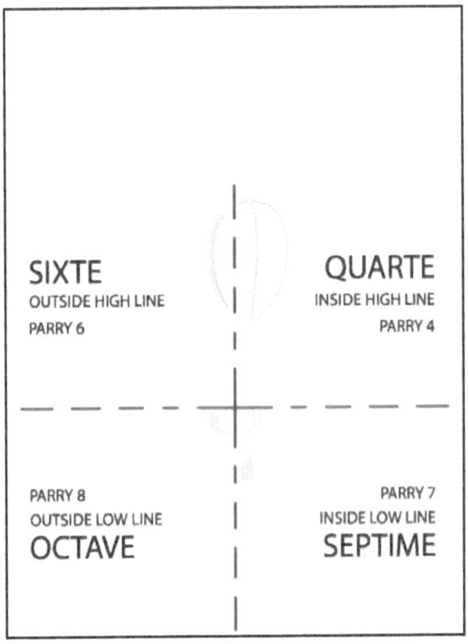


Figure 1

These two imaginary lines intersect where the blade meets the bell (figure 1) As you move your blade, the intersecting lines will move and adjust the parry zones. This will make one zone smaller and the opposing zone larger (Figure 2 below).

If this is done to the extreme where you completely close off one of the zones, it may cause you to over compensate with the opposing parry and lose control of the bout.

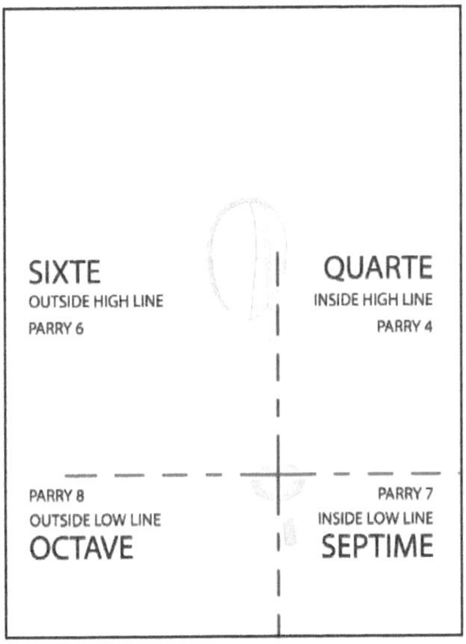


Figure 2

# PARRIES

Parry names and numbering have changed through the years. Every region and weapon has its own names and explanations for the parries. The thing to remember is the purpose of the parry: a defensive action made against the opponent's attack, which allows the fencer to render the attack null. This gives the defendant the opportunity to attack (Riposte).

There are two recognized schools of foil fencing: the French and the Italian. The French method is now generally adopted everywhere except in Italy. Parries described below are from the French school.

> Pronation - noun - rotation of the hand or forearm so that the surface of the palm is facing downward or toward the back (opposed to supination).
>
> http://dictionary.reference.com/browse/pronation

> Supination - noun - rotation of the hand or forearm so that the palm surface is facing upward (opposed to pronation).
>
> http://dictionary.reference.com/browse/supination

## Parry 4 (quarte)

- Start from an En Garde
- As an attack approaches your torso, roll your weapon hand toward the floor (supination) keeping your elbow bent
- Catch the foible (weak) of your opponent's blade with the forte (strong) of your blade, moving your opponent's blade out of line.

**Parry 6 (sixte)**

- Start from an En Garde
- As an attack approaches your torso, roll your weapon hand up toward the ceiling (pronation) keeping your elbow bent
- Catch the foible (weak) of your opponent's blade with the forte (strong) of your blade, moving your opponent's blade out of line.

---

**Parry 7 (septime)**

- Start from an En Garde
- As an attack approaches your torso, lower the tip of your blade toward the floor
- Roll your weapon hand toward the floor (supination) keeping your elbow bent
- Catch the foible (weak) of your opponent's blade with the forte (strong) of your blade, moving your opponent's blade out of line.

---

**Parry 8 (octave)**

- Start from an En Garde
- As an attack approaches your torso, lower the tip of your blade toward the floor
- Roll your weapon hand up toward the ceiling (pronation) keeping your elbow bent
- Catch the foible (weak) of your opponent's blade with the forte (strong) of your blade, moving your opponent's blade out of line.

# COUPÉ / DISENGAGE

## Feint

Feint is an offensive movement resembling an attack. You will attack into one line with the intention of switching to another line before the attack is completed. A Feint is designed to draw a reaction from an opponent. This is the 'intention'. The reaction is generally a parry and then you can follow with either a Coupé or a Disengage.

---

## Coupé

Coupé is where we get the English automotive term coup: a car with a fixed roof (top) and two doors. The Coupé, also called a Cut-Over, is an indirect attack following a Feint. The attacking blade is pulled up and over the opponent's parrying blade; typically a lower parry with the blade cut-over the top. This maneuver requires the twisting of the wrist only, since moving the entire arm and blade backwards would forfeit right-of-way. The Cut-Over retains right-of-way during its entire execution if: executed quickly, with good distance, and the point never moves backwards.

---

## Disengage

As with the Coupé, the Disengage also uses a Feint that is typically utilized with an extension/attack. To use Disengage in an attack, start with a Feint attack with an extension and avoid the opponent's attempt to parry or press your blade by making the smallest circular motion possible. Circling under the opponent's blade typically works best against upper parries. The first extension must be a believable Feint in order to draw a reaction. Be prepared to proceed forward with a straight attack if your opponent does not parry in response to the Feint.

**Derobement**

An offensive Derobement is when an opponent is attempting to take the blade without beginning an attack. This is done through either entrapping, beating or pressing in a circular, lateral, vertical or diagonal motion. A defensive Derobement is an avoidance of the entrapping, beating or pressing. This avoidance can be executed either by a Coupé or by a Disengage followed by your attack.

# SEMAPHORES

semə͵fôr/ noun

A system of sending messages by holding the arms, two flags or poles in certain positions according to an alphabetic (or other) code.

In classical and modern fencing, the Judge needs to indicate which actions were taken on the strip. The Judge will use what we call semaphores. These signals have a couple advantages:

1. In international tournaments, both opponents will know what call is made, without it having to be translated into their own spoken language.
2. People watching the match will also know what actions were accomplished.

The below semaphores have the Judge facing away from the reader, facing the strip.

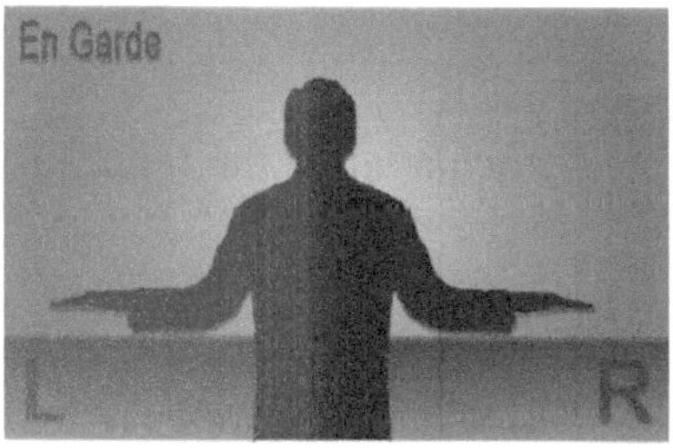


**En Garde**

First of three calls to start a bout

Arms out to the side with forearms parallel with the floor, palms down and elbows away from the body and bent just over 90 degrees

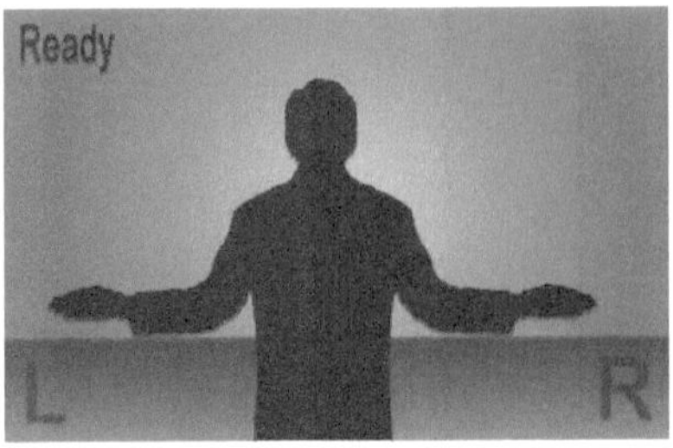


**Ready**
Second of three calls to start a bout

Arms out to the side with forearms parallel with the floor, palms facing the strip with elbows away from the body and bent just over 90 degrees

---

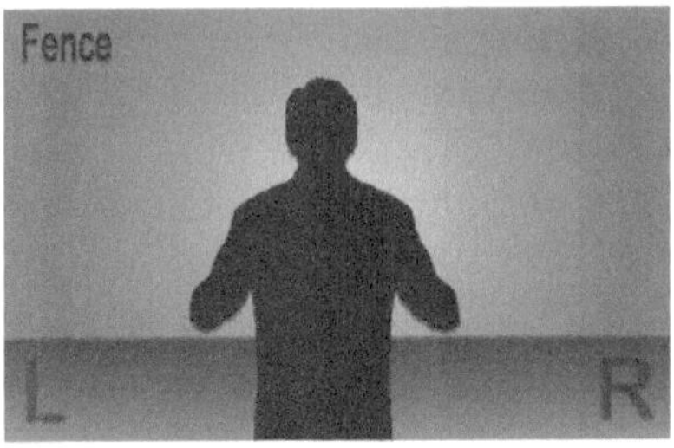


**Fence**
Third and final call to start the bout

From the "READY" stance, begin to bring both hands together, as if to clap, but hands stop once elbows and hands are inline straight out front

---

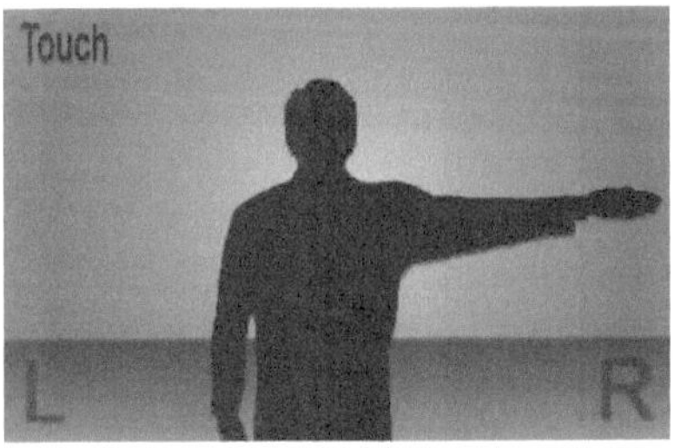


**Touch**
Touch against the fencer on the Right

Arm straight out from the shoulder with palm facing the strip

---

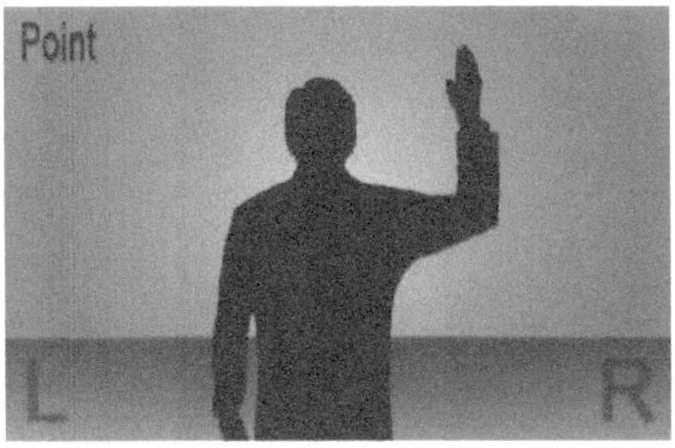


**Point**
Touch awarded to fencer on the Right

Elbow bent at 90 degrees, with upper arm parallel to the ground, palm facing the strip

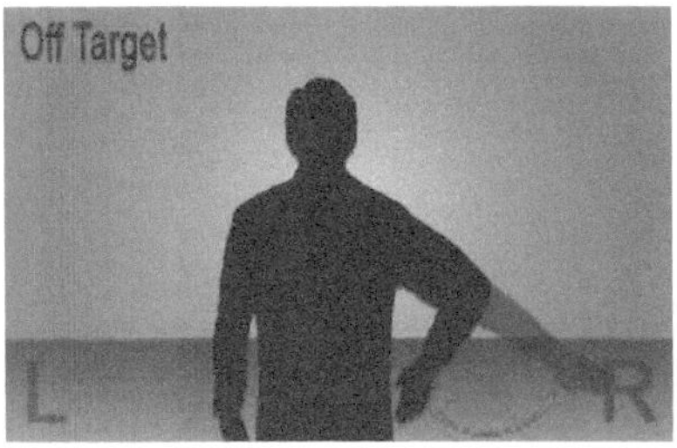


**Off Target**
Fencer to the Right lands off target

Upper arm at 45 degrees, palm facing away from the strip, swinging the forearm side-to-side

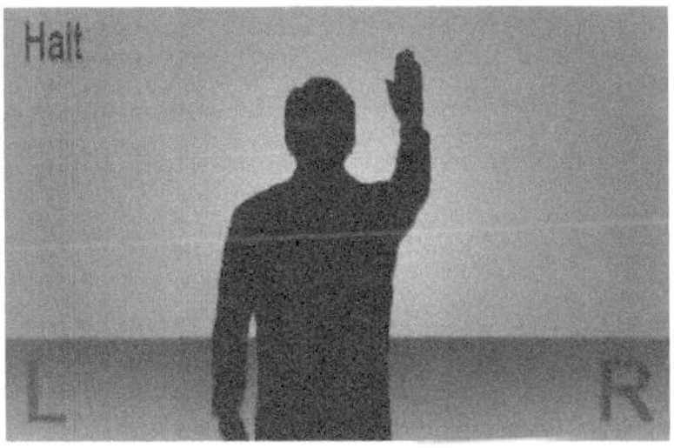


**Halt**
Called to stop a bout

Hand held directly out in front of the Judge, with palm facing the strip. If there is an infraction by one of the fencers, then it should be the hand on the side of that fencer raised

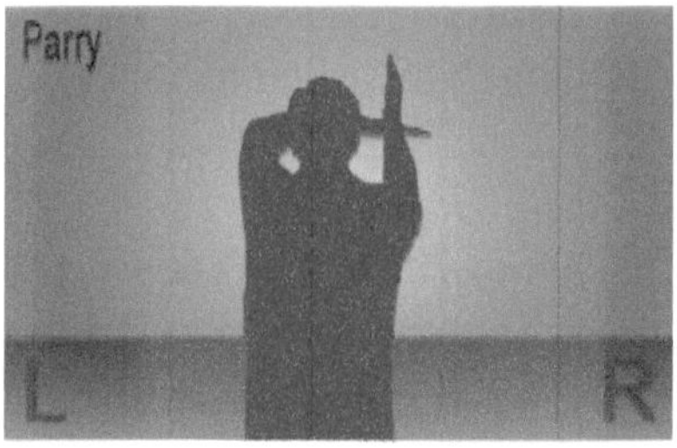


**Parry**
Fencer on the Right parries the attack that came from the fencer on the Left

The left arm is held in front of the face showing the attack, and the right arm comes up crossing over the left arm

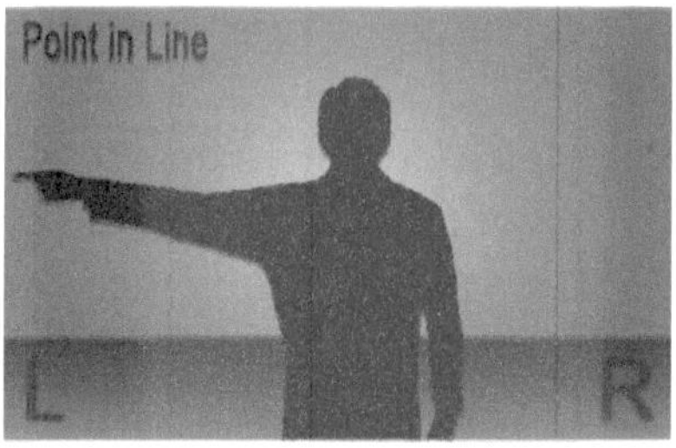


**Point in Line**
The fencer on the Right has established right-of-way

Arm straight out from the shoulder with the index finger extended

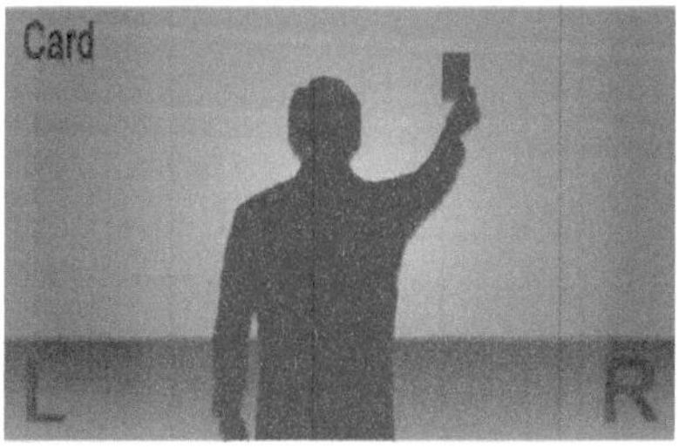


**Card**
Fencer Right has received a card for an illegal action

Card is held up in front of the Judge toward the fencer on the right

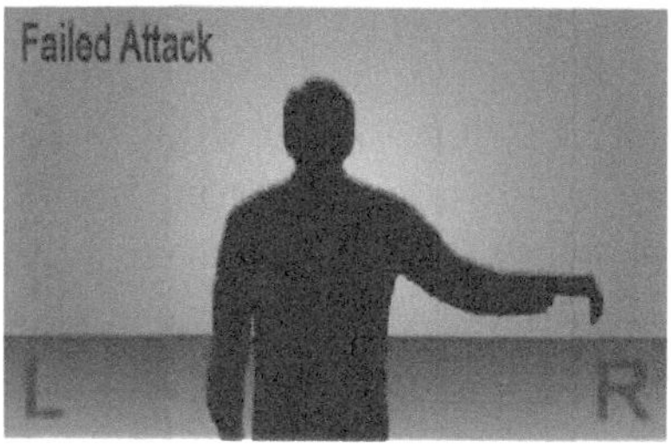


**Failed Attack**
Failed attack could be any of the following: stop-hit, counterattack, remise, reprise, etc.
Arm extended to the side of the failed attack with hand bent at 90 degrees, fingers pointing toward the ground

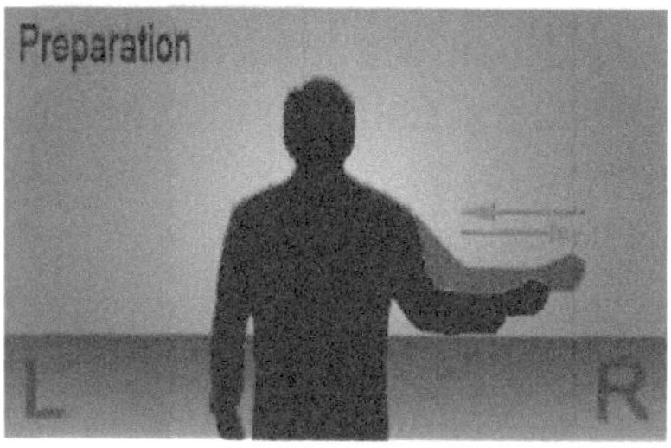


**Preparation**
The action from the Right does not qualify as an attack

The arm is bent at just over 90 degrees, with the hand in a fist, moving back and forth in a pumping action

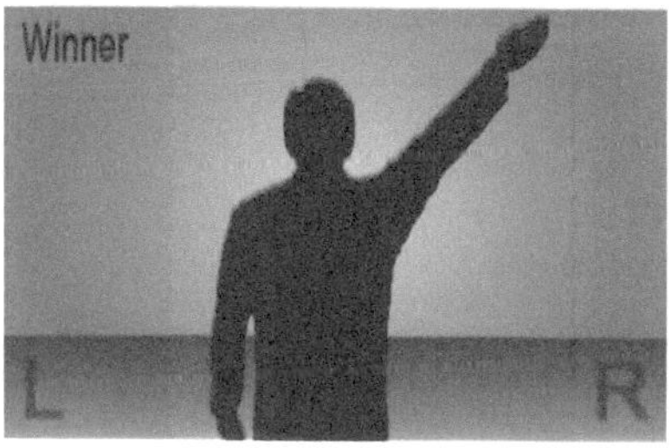


**Winner**
To award the match to the fencer on the Right

Arm straight out from the shoulder at about a 45 degree angle, palm facing the winner

## JUDGING A BOUT

In Classical Fencing, they may use up to five Judges for tournaments. You would have one President and four Jurors.

- The President is positioned in the center of the strip and is in control of the entire strip.
- The Jurors (A) are positioned around the strip, with two of the Jurors positioned just behind "Fencer Right", on both sides of the strip, and the other two behind "Fencer Left".

From these positions, the fencers can see all sides of the action. All Jurors and the President will move with the fencers as they advance and retreat on the strip.

Once the President calls "Halt" or "Stop" the entire group of the Jury will use the semaphores to let the President know what they have seen. Only the President will call halt, unless a Juror sees a safety issue.

The President will then award the touch and may recall the last few moves by using semaphores.

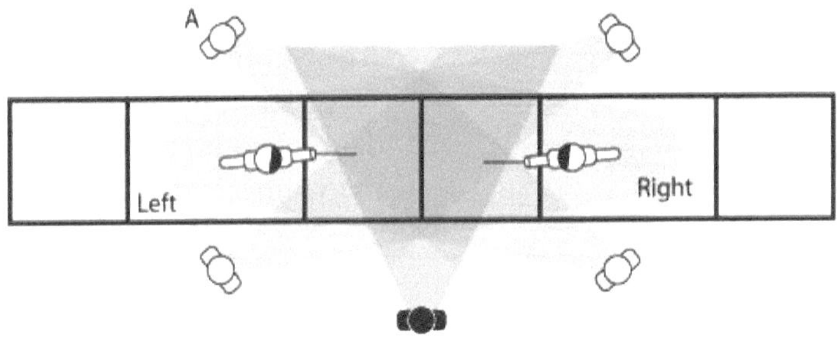

**Judging A Foil Fencing Bout**

Here are some judging techniques that are useful for Presidents during a Foil bout.

- Keep attention on the entire strip
  -That no one impedes the fencers, including participants or Jurors
- Use "Soft Focus" (Vision)
  - Look past the blades, taking in everything between "Fencer Left" and "Fencer Right"
- Foil is a right-of-way (priority) weapon
- Target area in Foil: torso only
- Once a fencer begins the attack, use full extension and forward motion (right-of-way), focusing down more on the blade, yet still using soft focus
- If not parried, then focus on the tip of the blade to see if the tip sets on target area. Call "HOLD" or "HALT" and award point
  OR
  If the attacking blade is parried, then follow the defending blade as it may take right-of-way, to see if tip is set on target area. Call "HOLD" or "HALT" and award point
- If the blade with right-of-way sets on a non-target area, call "HOLD" or "HALT", and continue the bout from the position the fencers were at when the action was halted
- If the blade with right-of-way misses the opponent entirely, then check the other fencer's tip. If it is set on target area, or off-target, call "HOLD" or "HALT" and award point, or continue the bout
- If both blades miss setting a point, then allow the bout to continue until one fencer sets a point. Call "HOLD" or "HALT" and award point

# APPENDIX A

## Equipment Safety

| Equipment | Description | Safety |
|---|---|---|
| Jacket (Minimum Required Equipment) | Form-fitting jacket includes: 1.”v” portion covering groin with strap between the legs. 2. “gorget” portion of folded fabric sewn around the jacket collar to prevent an opponent's blade from slipping under the mask upward towards the neck | Protects the torso, groin and neck |
| Mask (Minimum Required Equipment) | Includes a bib, which protects the neck. The mask can usually support 12 kilograms (26 lbs.) on the metal mesh and 350 newton (79 lbs.) of penetration resistance on the bib. FIE regulations dictate that masks must withstand 25 kilograms (55 lbs.) on the mesh and 1,600 Newton (360 lbs.) on the bib | Protects the entire face and neck from any direct hit |

| **Equipment** | **Description** | **Safety** |
|---|---|---|
| Glove | One glove with a gauntlet for the weapon hand protecting the hand and providing a good grip | The gauntlet prevents blades from going up the sleeve |
| Plastron | An underarm protector, which goes underneath the jacket | Provides double protection on the sword arm side and upper arm |
| Knickers | A pair of short trousers that end just below the knee. The breeches are required to have 10 cm of overlap with the jacket. Most are equipped with suspenders | |
| Socks | Knee-high socks, which cover knee and thighs just above the knee. Soccer style socks work well | |

| Equipment | Description | Safety |
|---|---|---|
| Shoes (Minimum Required Equipment) | Flat soles with low profile heel and with good traction | Good grip to prevent sliding |
| Chest Protector | One eighth inch thick plastic protector form-fitted to the body | Mandatory for females during competition |

# APPENDIX B

## *GLOSSARY OF FENCING TERMS*

**Advance:**
a forward movement performed by a fencer on the strip

**Attack:**
the initial attack made by extending the sword arm and threatening a valid target area of your opponent

**Balestra:**
a forward jump, followed by a lunge to cover a large distance

**Black Card:**
the final penalty for the most serious offenses in a fencing bout, followed by the expulsion of the offending fencer from the event

**Bout:**
two fencers engaged in opposition with scores being tallied

**Button:**
also known as "tip": the safety tip on the end of a practice foil blade

**Compound:**
an attack with two or more movements

**Counter-attack:**
an attack made against your opponent's right-of-way attack

**Corps-a-corps:**
"body-to-body"; physical contact of two fencers during a bout which may or may not incur a penalty dependent on situation

**Cross:**
an advance or retreat by crossing one leg over the other, with feet staying in proper alignment

**Disengage:**
a circular movement of the blade that deceives the opponent's parry

**En Garde:**
also "On Guard": a fencing position used to begin a bout; A.K.A. "First Position"

**Feint:**
an attack into one line with the intention of switching to another line before the attack is completed

**Foible:**
the weak part of the fencing blade

**Foil:**
a fencing blade with a small bell guard. Foil also means to "fold over" to make less dangerous

**Forte:**
the strong part of the fencing blade

**Guard:**
the metal cup on the fencing foil that protects the hand from being hit; also used defensively in parries

**Jury:**
4 officials who watch for hits in a dry (non-electric) fencing bout

**Lunge:**
a main attack performed by extending the weapon while pushing off with the back foot and landing on the front foot with knee bent at 90 degrees. This is also known as "Second Position"

**Measure:**
the distance between two fencers

**Octave:**
parry #8; blade down and to the outside, wrist supinated

**Parry:**
a diverting of an attack, made with the forte (strong) of your fencing blade

**Passe':**
an attack that passes by the target area on the opponent

**Phrase:**
a set of related actions and reactions in a fencing bout

**Piste:**
A.K.A., "strip" on which a fencing bout takes place; measures approximately 2m x 14m

**Pistol Grip:**
a modern, ergonomic grip. Varying styles/fits of pistol grips include: Belgian, German, Russian, and Visconti

**Point:**
a valid touch on an opponent's target area

**Point-in-Line:**
an extended fencing blade and arm, targeting a valid target area

**Pommel:**
a weighted fastener that holds the fencing blade together

**Quarte:**
Parry #4; blade up and to the inside, wrist supinated

**Red Card:**
the penalty for a minor offense or a major rule infraction by a fencer, resulting in a point awarded to the other fencer. Multiple red cards can be issued, resulting in multiple points awarded to the other fencer

**Referee:**
A.K.A. Director or President who watches for touches and keeps score of the fencing bout

**Remise:**
immediate replacement/continuance of an attack that was either missed or parried, without withdrawing the arm

**Retreat:**
step back; opposite of advance

**Right-of-way:**
To gain right-of-way, one must have "Point-in-Line" together with forward motion. Right-of-way determines which opponent has the right to score in a foil or saber fencing bout

**Riposte:**
an attack you make immediately after parrying your opponent's attack

**Salute:**
a motion made with the fencing foil, acknowledging your opponent and referee at the start and end of the fencing bout

**Septime:**
parry #7; blade down and to the inside, wrist supinated

**Simultaneous:**
both opponents attacking at the same time, causing the right-of-way to be too close to determine

**Sixte:**
parry #6; blade up and to the outside, wrist supinated

**Supinated:**
wrist and palm turned upward, as in parries 4 and 7

**Thrust:**
an attack made by moving the sword and arm in full extension

**Touch:**
may or may not score a point, depending upon whether it is or is not on a valid target area of your opponent

**Yellow Card:**

used to indicate a minor rule infraction in a fencing bout and given without a point awarded to the other fencer

# APPENDIX C

## PARTIAL LIST OF FEELING WORDS

For help with the feeling Formula in the Values Worksheets.

Abandoned
Accepted
Aggressive
Alienated
Amazed
Amused
Anxious
Apathetic
Ashamed
Astonished
Aversion
Avoidance
Awed
Awful
Bored
Confident
Confused
Courageous
Critical
Depressed
Despair
Detestable
Devastated
Disappointed
Disapproving
Disillusioned
Dismayed
Disrespectful
Distant
Eager
Ecstatic
Embarrassed
Empty
Energetic
Enraged
Excited
Frightened
Frustrated
Fulfilled
Furious
Guilty
Hateful
Hesitant
Hopeful
Hostile
Humiliated
Hurt
Ignored
Important
Inadequate
Indifferent
Inferior
Infuriated
Inquisitive
Insecure
Insignificant
Inspired
Interested
Intimate
Irritated
Isolated
Jealous
Joyful
Judgmental
Liberated
Loathing
Lonely
Open
Loving
Mad
Optimistic
Overwhelmed
Peaceful
Perplexed
Playful
Powerful
Powerless
Proud
Provoked
Rejected
Rebuffed
Remorseful
Repugnant
Resentful
Respected
Receiving
Ridicule
Sarcastic
Scared
Sensitive
Shocked
Skeptical
Startled
Submissive
Suspicious
Terrified
Threatened
Victimized
Vulnerable
Withdrawn
Worried
Worthless

# KNIGHTLY VALUES WORKSHEETS

## COMPASSION WORKSHEET

What is your personal definition of Compassion?

Is having compassion for others easy for you? Yes No
Why?

**This week's challenge:** take time to observe people and make notes on how you felt about things such as: their actions, situation, appearance, what they talked about, or where you saw them.

# KINDNESS WORKSHEET

What is your personal definition of Kindness?

On a scale of 1 to 10 (10 being greatest)
What is your Kindness Level?
1 2 3 4 5 6 7 8 9 10

What things could you do to practice more kindness?

**This week's challenge:** show kindness (examples: being polite, giving, appreciation, consideration), to three people: One adult, one classmate and one person younger than you. Write what you did for them.

# HUMILITY WORKSHEET

What is your personal definition of Humility?

Is it easy for you to walk in Humility? Yes No
Why?

**This week's challenge:** see where you can put someone else's needs first without letting him or her know and write about your experience here.

# QUIET STRENGTH WORKSHEET

What is your personal definition of Quiet Strength?

Name three people you know who have lived out Quiet Strength in one way or another.

**This week's challenge:** look for the opportunity to walk out the value of quiet strength. Take time to write down the situation and how God is helping you to walk out quiet strength.

# DISCIPLINE WORKSHEET

What is your personal definition of Discipline?

______________________________________________

______________________________________________

______________________________________________

______________________________________________

**This week's challenge:** observe and write down the people around you who are walking in the character values you want in your life.

______________________________________________

______________________________________________

______________________________________________

______________________________________________

______________________________________________

______________________________________________

Take time to talk with that person and ask them to be your mentor.

**The Best Mentor Ever**
If you have not yet asked Jesus to be the Lord of your life and received the Holy Spirit to be your mentor, talk with the person who gave you this book and pray the following prayer.

> **Prayer:**
> *God I know that Jesus Christ came as a man, died on the cross for my failures and shortcomings (sin), rose from the grave and sits with you in heaven. I accept Jesus Christ as my Lord and Savior and ask Him and the Holy Spirit to be my mentor.*

# EVEN-TEMPERED WORKSHEET

What is your personal definition of Even-Tempered?

________________________________________

________________________________________

________________________________________

________________________________________

How do you deal with your feelings?

________________________________________

________________________________________

________________________________________

**This week's challenge:** Use the Feeling Formula below to properly deal with your feelings. Take time and talk with your mentor about these feelings.

I FEEL __________________________________<br>
ABOUT __________________________________<br>
BECAUSE ________________________________

Rules for I FEEL

- Use only emotional words in the feeling area
- Do not use LIKE "I Feel Like…"

Rules for About

- Do not use a person's name in the about area; if that person never changes you will never be able to resolve your feelings.

Rules for BECAUSE

- Start by using a phrase "I think" or "I am".
- This could bring up other feeling words that you might have to work through in another Feeling Formula.

Once you have the "BECAUSE" this is typically, what we call your ungodly belief or untruth. You have to replace that ungodly belief with what God is saying about you: Godly Belief or the truth. Take this ungodly belief to God in prayer and ask Him what He says about you.

Then search the Bible to find scriptures that confirm these new Godly Beliefs, and begin to recite the Godly Beliefs and scriptures for the next 21 days.

Feeling Formula is a tool we received from Paraklesis Ministries - Dave and Linda Roeder. For more information on their ministry and resources see www.dave-linda.com

# CONTENT WORKSHEET

What is your personal definition of Content?

Where does true contentment come from?

**This week's challenge:** take note and write down three areas in your life that you feel contentment in and why.

# FORGIVENESS WORKSHEET

What is your personal definition of Forgiveness?

______________________________________________

______________________________________________

______________________________________________

| | | |
|---|---|---|
| Do you have memories that are still painful to recall? | **Yes** | **No** |
| Are you ready to forgive? | **Yes** | **No** |

**This lifelong challenge:** If yes to the above questions, pray this simple prayer of forgiveness. *[Scripture listed below]*

*Lord, I thank you for the power of forgiveness, and I choose to forgive ____________________ who has hurt me, for the offense of ______________________________. I leave these offenses at the foot of the cross. I release them to You [Romans 12:19]. Help me bless those who have hurt me [Romans 12:14]. Help me walk in righteousness, peace, and joy. I choose to be kind and compassionate, forgiving others, just as You forgave me [Ephesians 4:32]. In Jesus' name, amen.*

> Romans 12:19 (NIV) "Do not take revenge, my dear friends, but leave room for God's wrath, for it is written: "It is mine to avenge; I will repay," says the Lord."
>
> Romans 12:14 (NIV) "Bless those who persecute you; bless and do not curse."
>
> Ephesians 4:32 (NIV) "Be kind and compassionate to one another, forgiving each other, just as in Christ God forgave you."